PALLIATIVE CARE, MUSCULOSKELETAL CONDITIONS, PRESCRIBING PRACTICE

Gill Wakley
Ruth Chambers
and
Clare Gerada

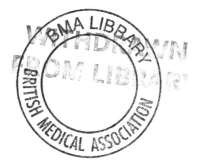

RADCLIFFE PUBLISHING
Oxford • Seattle

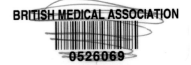

Radcliffe Publishing Ltd
18 Marcham Road
Abingdon
Oxon OX14 1AA
United Kingdom

www.radcliffe-oxford.com
Electronic catalogue and worldwide online ordering facility.

_____

British Library Cataloguing in Publication Data

A catalogue record for this book is available from the British Library.

ISBN 1 85775 614 2

Typeset by Advance Typesetting Ltd, Oxford
Printed and bound by T J International, Padstow, Cornwall

Contents

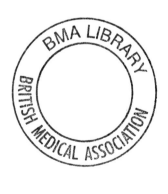

Preface

The General Medical Council has asked doctors to start thinking now about how they will collect and keep the information that will show that they should continue to hold a licence to practise as doctors from 2005 onwards. The onus will be on individual doctors to show that they are up to date and fit to practise medicine throughout their careers. It will be doctors who decide for themselves the nature of the information they collect and retain that best reflects their roles and responsibilities in their everyday work.

This book is one of a series that will guide you as a general practitioner (GP) though the process, giving you examples and ideas as to how to document your learning, competence, performance or standards of service delivery. At the same time as you are collecting the data to demonstrate your own competence, you are also helping to show that your practice is achieving high standards of care. The quality points available from the quality and outcomes framework of the General Medical Services (GMS) contract for general practice are achievable on a sliding scale.[1] As you increase your knowledge and skills in the clinical fields covered by the contract and improve your practice organisation with service developments, you should be working towards maximising your quality points. Some of the quality indicators are generic to various clinical areas such as smoking status, smoking cessation advice and influenza immunisation, and obviously overlap. Others such as good record keeping, consistent approach to maintaining disease registers, medicines management and education/appraisal of staff should underpin all the clinical areas. As we cover the clinical topics in this book in Chapters 5 to 11, we point out what quality points are available in that clinical area. Other books in the series also include clinical topics within the scope of the GMS contract – so it will be useful for you to read them too (e.g. coronary heart disease and stroke are included in: Wakley G, Chambers R and Ellis S (2004) *Demonstrating Your Competence 3: Cardiovascular and Neurological Conditions*. Radcliffe Publishing, Oxford).

Chapter 1 explains the link between your personal development plans, local appraisal and the revalidation of your medical registration. Learning and service improvements that are integral to your personal development plan are central to the evidence you include in your appraisal and revalidation portfolio.

The stages of the evidence cycle that we suggest are built upon the underpinning publication: Chambers R, Wakley G, Field S and Ellis S (2002) *Appraisal for the Apprehensive*. Radcliffe Medical Press, Oxford.

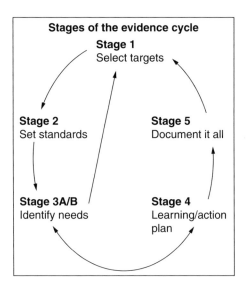

Stage 1 is about setting targets or aspirations for good practice. Many of the aspirations we suggest are taken from *Good Medical Practice* or its sister publication, *Good Medical Practice for General Practitioners*.[2,3] Stage 2 encourages you, as a doctor, to set standards for the outcomes of what you plan to learn more about, or outcomes relating to you providing a good service in your practice.

Chapter 2 describes a variety of methods to help you to address Stage 3 of the cycle of evidence, to find out what it is you need to learn about or what gaps there are in the way you deliver care as an individual GP or as a team. This chapter includes a wide variety of methods doctors might use in their everyday work to identify and document these needs. One of the drivers for the introduction of appraisal and revalidation has been to reassure the public and others of doctors' continuing fitness to practise. So it makes sense that we have emphasised the importance of obtaining feedback from patients in this chapter in relation to identifying your learning and service development needs.

Best practice in addressing the giving of informed consent by patients, maintaining confidentiality of patient information and organising responsive complaints processes are all common components of good quality healthcare. Chapter 3 covers these aspects in depth and provides the first example of cycles of evidence for you to consider adopting or adapting for your own circumstances. The focus of each cycle of evidence is on one of the 'headings' from *Good Medical Practice*[2] or standard appraisal format.

Chapter 4 gives you information about what is required of a GP with a special interest, taking drug abuse as an example. The rest of the book consists of clinically based chapters that span key clinical topics. The first part of each chapter covers key issues that are likely to crop up in typical consultations for each clinical field. The second part of each chapter gives examples of cycles of evidence in a similar format to those in Chapter 3.

Overall, you will probably want to choose three or four cycles of evidence each year. You might choose one or two from Chapter 3 and the rest from clinical areas such as those covered by the later chapters. You might like this way of learning and service development so much that you build up a bigger bank of evidence, taking one cycle from each chapter in the same year. Whatever your approach, you will want to keep your cycles of evidence as short and simple as possible, so that the documentation itself is a by-product of the learning and action plans you undertake to improve the service you provide, and does not dominate your time and effort at work.

Other books in the series are based on the same format of the five stages in the cycle of evidence. Book 1 helps doctors and other health professionals to demonstrate that they are competent teachers or trainers, and Books 2, 3 and 4 set out key information and examples of evidence for a wide variety of clinical areas for GPs and other doctors.

This approach and style of learning will take a bit of getting used to for doctors. Until now, they have not had to prove that they are fit to practise unless the General Medical Council has investigated them for a significant reason such as a complaint or error. Until recently, most doctors did not evaluate what they learnt or whether they applied it in practice. They did not protect time for learning and reflection among their everyday responsibilities, or target their time and effort on priority topics. Times are changing, and with the introduction of personal development plans and appraisal, GPs are realising that they must take a more professional approach to learning, and document their standards of competence, performance and service delivery. This book helps them to do just that.

Please note that resources to support this book are provided at http://health.mattersonline.net.

References

1   General Practitioners Committee/The NHS Confederation (2003) *New GMS Contract. Investing in general practice*. General Practitioners Committee/NHS Confederation, London.

2   General Medical Council (2001) *Good Medical Practice*. General Medical Council, London.

3   Royal College of General Practitioners/General Practitioners Committee (2002) *Good Medical Practice for General Practitioners*. Royal College of General Practitioners, London.

About the authors

Gill Wakley started in general practice but transferred to community medicine shortly afterwards and then into public health. A desire for increased contact with patients caused a move back into general practice. She has been heavily involved in learning and teaching throughout her career. She was in a training general practice, became an instructing doctor and a regional assessor in family planning, and was until recently a senior clinical lecturer with the Primary Care Department at Keele University. Like Ruth, she has run all types of educational initiatives and activities. A visiting professor at Staffordshire University, she now works as a freelance GP, writer and lecturer.

Ruth Chambers has been a GP for more than 20 years and is currently the head of the Stoke-on-Trent Teaching Primary Care Trust programme and professor of primary care development at Staffordshire University. Ruth has worked with the Royal College of General Practitioners to enable GPs to gather evidence about their learning and standards of practice while striving to be excellent GPs. Ruth has co-authored a series of books with Gill, designed to help readers draw up their own personal development plans or workplace learning plans around key clinical topics.

Clare Gerada has been a GP in a South London practice for 14 years and previously trained as a psychiatrist at the Maudsley Hospital. She has a special interest in drug misuse and leads the Royal College of General Practitioners (RCGP) drug misuse training programme. She has worked in the Department of Health in various guises for a number of years, and is currently Director of Primary Care for the Clinical Governance Support Team. She has published widely on a number of topics related to drug and alcohol problems, primary care and clinical governance. She led the RCGP development of the Frameworks for General Practitioners with Special Interests.

1

Making the link: personal development plans, appraisal and revalidation

The nexus of personal development plans, appraisal and revalidation

Learning involves many steps. It includes the acquisition of information, its retention, the ability to retrieve the information when needed and how to use that information for best practice. Demonstrating your learning involves being able to show the steps you have taken. Learning should be lifelong and encompass continuing professional development.

Continuing professional development (CPD) takes time. It makes sense to utilise the time spent by overlapping learning to meet your personal and professional needs with that required for the performance of your role in the health service.

Many doctors have drawn up a personal development plan (PDP) that is agreed with their local CPD or college tutor. Some doctors have constructed their PDP in a systematic way and identified the priorities within it, or gathered evidence to demonstrate that what they learnt about was subsequently applied in practice. Tutors do not have a uniform approach to the style and relevance of a doctor's PDP. Some are content that a plan has been drawn up, while others encourage the doctor to develop a systematic approach to identifying and addressing their learning and service needs, in order of importance or urgency.[1]

The new emphasis on doctors' accountability to the public has given the PDP a higher profile and shown that it may be used in other ways. The medical education establishment and NHS management argue about the balance between its alternative uses. The educationalists view a PDP as a tool to encourage doctors to plan their own learning activities. The management view is of a tool allowing quality assurance of the doctor's performance. Doctors, striving to improve the quality of the care that they deliver to patients, want to use a PDP to guide them on their way, perhaps towards postgraduate awards of universities or the quality awards of the Royal College of General Practitioners. These quality awards are built around the standards of excellence to which a general practitioner (GP) should aspire, as described in the publication, *Good Medical Practice for General Practitioners*.[2]

Your personal development plan

Your PDP will be an integral part of your future appraisal and revalidation portfolio to demonstrate your fitness to practise as a doctor.

Your initial plan should:

- identify your gaps or weaknesses in knowledge, skills or attitudes
- specify topics for learning as a result of changes: in your role, responsibilities, the organisation in which you work
- link into the learning needs of others in your workplace or team of colleagues
- tie in with the service development priorities of your practice, the primary care organisation (PCO) or the NHS as a whole
- describe how you identified your learning needs
- set your learning needs and associated goals in order of importance and urgency
- justify your selection of learning goals
- describe how you will achieve your goals and over what time period
- describe how you will evaluate learning outcomes.

Each year you will continue or revise your PDP. It should demonstrate how you carried out your learning and evaluation plans, show that you have learnt what you set out to do (or why it was modified) and how you applied your new learning in practice. In addition, you will find that you have new priorities and fresh learning needs as circumstances change.

The main task is to capture what you have learnt, in a way that suits you. Then you can look back at what you have done and:

- reflect on it later, to decide to learn more, or to make changes as a result, and identify further needs
- demonstrate to others that you are fit to practise or work through:
  - what you have done
  - what you have learnt
  - what changes you have made as a result
  - the standards of work you have achieved and are maintaining
  - how you monitor your performance at work

- use it to show how your personal learning fits in with the requirements of your practice or the NHS, and other people's personal and professional development plans.

Organise all the evidence of your learning into a CPD portfolio of some sort. It is up to you how you keep this record of your learning. Examples are:

- *an ongoing learning journal* in which you draw up and describe your plan, record how you determined your needs and prioritised them, report why you attended particular educational meetings or courses and what you got out of them as well as the continuing cycle of review, making changes and evaluating them
- *an A4 file* with lots of plastic sleeves into which you build up a systematic record of your educational activities in line with your plan
- *a box*: chuck in everything to do with your learning plan as you do it and sort it out into a sensible order every few months with a good review once a year.

The context of appraisal and revalidation

Appraisal and revalidation are based on the same sources of information – presented in the same structure as the headings set out in the General Medical Council (GMC) guidance in *Good Medical Practice*.[3] The two processes perform different functions. Whereas revalidation involves an assessment against a standard of fitness to practise medicine, appraisal is concerned with the doctor's professional development within his or her working environment and the needs of the organisation for which the doctor works.

Appraisal is a formative and developmental process that is being introduced by the Departments of Health for all GPs and hospital consultants working in the NHS across the UK. While the details of the appraisal system vary for consultants and GPs and for each of the countries, the educational principles remain the same. The aims of the appraisal system are to give doctors an opportunity to discuss and receive regular feedback on their previous and continuing performance and identify education and development needs.

The drive to introduce formal appraisals came initially as part of the programme to introduce clinical governance across the NHS as laid out in the 1998 consultation document *A First Class Service*.[4] Momentum was gained with the publication of *Supporting Doctors, Protecting Patients* (1999) in England which outlined a set of proposals to help prevent doctors from developing problems.[5] Appraisal was at the heart of the proposals as:

a positive process to give someone feedback on their performance, to chart their continuing progress and to identify development needs. It is a forward looking process essential for the developmental and educational planning needs of an individual. *Assessment* is the process of measuring progress against agreed criteria.... It is not the primary aim of appraisal to scrutinise doctors to see if they are performing poorly but rather to help them consolidate and improve on good performance aiming towards excellence.[5]

The document went on to suggest that appraisal should be made comprehensive and compulsory for doctors working in the NHS and form part of a future revalidation system.

In addition, appraisal should also address other areas of particular importance to the individual doctor. A standardised approach has been developed that utilises approved documentation. This should ensure that information from a variety of NHS employers is recorded consistently. The format of the paperwork is slightly different for consultants and GPs.

Appraisal must be a positive, formative and developmental process to support high quality patient care and improve clinical standards. Appraisal is different from, but linked to, revalidation.[6] Revalidation is the process whereby doctors will be regularly required to demonstrate that they are fit to practise. Appraisal feeds into this by contributing to the information that a doctor supplies for the revalidation process. Appraisal will provide a regular structured recording system for documenting progress towards revalidation and identifying needs as part of the doctor's PDPs. Both the NHS appraisal and the revalidation structures are based on the same seven headings set out in the GMC's guidance *Good Medical Practice*.[3] The GMC claims, therefore, that 'five satisfactory appraisals equals revalidation'.[6] The GMC has also pledged that doctors not taking part in appraisal will be able to provide their own information for revalidation, providing this evidence meets the same criteria as in *Good Medical Practice*.

Appraisal is, however, a two-way process. Not only time, but also resources will be needed to make appraisal systems successful. In addition, appraisal will identify issues that will require extra investment by the NHS in the educational and organisational infrastructure.

Appraisal and revalidation processes are being increasingly integrated. The PDP is a central part of the appraisal documentation, which will in turn be included in the portfolio of information available for revalidation. It seems that the evolution will continue so that revalidation is met by supporting the appraisal documentation with additional documents about clinical governance activity and CPD. These supporting documents will be a mix of subjective and objective information that will include doctors' self-assessment of their performance and other work-based assessment.

The revalidation and appraisal processes need to be quality assured to be able to demonstrate that they can protect the public from poor or under-performing doctors. Such quality assurance will relate to the appraisers, their training and support, as well as systems to examine the quality of evidence in the documentation relating to a doctor's performance and outcomes of their PDP. You should regard your PDP and supporting documentation as central to the way in which you can show, to anyone who requires you to do so, that your performance as a doctor is acceptable and that you are trying to improve, or striving for excellence.

Demonstrating the standards of your practice

The GMC sets out standards that must be met as part of the duties and responsibilities of doctors in the booklet *Good Medical Practice*.[3] Doctors must be able to meet these standards with a record of their own performance in their revalidation portfolio if they want to retain a licence to practise. The nine key headings of expected standards of practice for all GPs working in England are shown in Box 1.1.

Box 1.1:   Key headings of expected standards of practice for GPs working in England

1 *Good professional practice.* This relates to clinical care, keeping records (including writing reports and keeping colleagues informed), access and availability, treatment in emergencies and making effective use of resources.
2 *Maintaining good medical practice.* This includes keeping up to date and maintaining your performance.
3 *Relationships with patients.* This encompasses providing information about your services, maintaining trust, avoiding discrimination and prejudice against patients, relating well to patients and apologising if things go wrong.
4 *Working with colleagues.* This relates to working with colleagues, working in teams, referring patients and accepting posts.
5 *Teaching and training, appraising and assessing.* You may be in a position to teach or train colleagues or students, and appraise or assess peers, employees or students.
6 *Probity* includes providing true information about your services, honesty in financial and commercial dealings, and providing references.
7 *Health* can include how you overcome or compensate for health problems in yourself, or help with or address health problems in other doctors.
8 *Research.* Conducting research in an ethical manner.
9 *Management.* The section on management concerns any responsibility GPs have for management outside the practice. GPs might wish to include management responsibilities that cross the interface between their practice and PCO.

The appraisal paperwork for GPs working in England, Scotland, Wales and Northern Ireland has been individualised by each country. The English version, for example, includes two extra sections to those of hospital consultants – management and research. The Scottish version focuses on core categories in preparation for revalidation of prescribing, referrals and peer review, clinical audit, significant event analysis and communication skills, summary of any complaints and other feedback.

The stages of the evidence cycle for demonstrating your standards of practice or competence and any necessary improvements are given in Figure 1.1. The stages of the evidence cycle are common to all the various areas of expertise considered in this book and will be followed in each chapter.

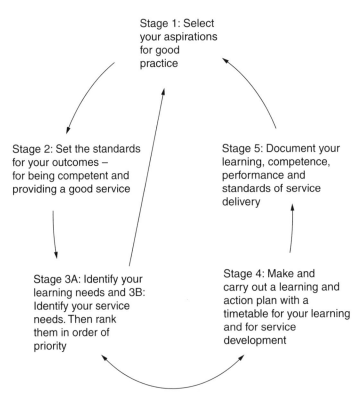

Stage 1: Select your aspirations for good practice

Stage 2: Set the standards for your outcomes – for being competent and providing a good service

Stage 5: Document your learning, competence, performance and standards of service delivery

Stage 3A: Identify your learning needs and 3B: Identify your service needs. Then rank them in order of priority

Stage 4: Make and carry out a learning and action plan with a timetable for your learning and for service development

Figure 1.1:   Stages of the evidence cycle.

Although the five stages are shown in sequence here, in practice you would expect to move backwards and forwards from stage to stage, because of new information or a modification of your earlier ideas. New information might accrue when research is published which affects your clinical behaviour or standards, or a critical incident or patient complaint might occur which causes you and others to think anew about your standards or the way that services are delivered. The arrows in Figure 1.1 show that you might re-set your target or aspirations for good practice having undertaken exercises to identify what you need to learn or determine if there are gaps in service delivery.

We suggest that you demonstrate your competence in focused areas of your day-to-day work by completing several cycles of evidence drawn from a variety of clinical or other areas each year, with at least one cycle of evidence from each of the main headings of *Good Medical Practice* over a five-year cycle.[3] By demonstrating your standards of practice around the main sections of *Good Medical Practice*, you will document your competence and performance for your revalidation portfolio in the same format as that required for your appraisal paperwork.

As you start to collate information about this five-stage cycle, discuss any problems about the standards of care or services you are looking at, with colleagues, experts in this area, tutors, etc. You want to develop a wide range and depth of evidence so that you can show that you are competent in your day-to-day general work as well as for any special areas of expertise.

Professional competence is the first area of concern in *Good Medical Practice*.[3] You should be able to demonstrate that you can maintain a satisfactory standard of clinical care most of the time in your everyday work. Some of the time you will be brilliant, of course! Celebrate those moments. On other occasions, you or others will be critical of your performance and feel that you could have done much better. Reflect on those episodes to learn from them.

Stage 1: Select your aspirations for good practice

By adopting or adapting descriptions of what an 'excellent' GP should be aiming for, you are defining the standards of practice for which all doctors should be aiming. The medical Royal Colleges have interpreted *Good Medical Practice* in various ways for the specialties of their own members.[3] For example, *Good Medical Practice for General Practitioners* describes the standards of practice that should be achieved by 'excellent' or 'unacceptable' GPs.[2] Their definition of excellence is being 'consistently good'.

This consistency is a critical factor in considering competence and performance too (*see* page 16). The documents that you collect in your evidence cycles must reflect consistency over time and in different circumstances, for example with various types of patients or your practice at different times of day. This will show that you have not only performed well on one occasion or for one type of baseline assessment, but also sustained your performance over time and under different conditions.

Stage 2: Set the standards of your outcomes – for being competent and providing a good service

Outcomes might include:

- the way that learning is applied
- a learnt skill
- a protocol
- a strategy that is implemented
- meeting recommended standards.

The level at which you should be performing depends on your particular field of expertise. GPs are good at seeing the wider picture, while specialists tend to be expert in a narrow area, so that the level of competence expected for a clinical area will vary depending on the doctor's role and responsibilities. You would not, for example, expect orthopaedic specialists to be competent at managing cardiac failure (although some of them may be), but you would expect GPs be able to manage all but the most complicated situations involving cardiac failure. You would expect both the orthopaedic specialist and the GP to recognise the limits of their competence and to refer to someone with more expertise when necessary.

Other standards include using resources effectively and the record keeping that is an essential tool in clinical care. As a health professional, you need to be accessible and available so that you can provide your services, and make suitable arrangements for handing over care to others. You must provide care in an emergency.

You could incorporate into your standards or outcomes those components specified by universities at a national level as part of their Masters Frameworks for their postgraduate awards. The Masters Frameworks consist of eight components that shape the individual postgraduate award programme outcomes and the learning outcomes of the individual modules for the postgraduate awards. The eight components are shown in Box 1.2. You could set out your CPD work in the portfolio you are assembling for revalidation and your annual appraisals in this format. This would help you to document your professional development to date in a form that can be readily 'accredited for prior experiential learning' (APEL) by universities (contact your local universities if you want more information about this process). You might then be given credits for learning against an intended postgraduate award. It would save you from duplicating work as well as speeding your progress through the award.

Box 1.2:   The eight components of the Masters Frameworks for postgraduate awards

1   Analysis
2   Problem solving
3   Knowledge and understanding
4   Reflection
5   Communication
6   Learning
7   Application
8   Enquiry

If you have information or data about your practice showing that it was substandard or that you were not competent, you might choose to exclude that from your portfolio. However, you will be able to show that you have learnt more by reviewing mistakes or negative episodes. It is better to include everything of relevance, then go on to demonstrate how you addressed the gaps in your performance and made sustained improvements. You will need to protect the confidentiality of patients and colleagues as necessary when you collect data. The GMC will be seeing the contents of your revalidation portfolio if your submission is one of those sampled. You will probably also submit or share the documentation for appraisal and maybe use it for reviews with colleagues or the PCO.

Stage 3: Identify your learning and service needs in your practice or primary care organisation and rank them in order of priority[1]

The type and depth of documentation you need to gather will encompass:

- the context in which you work
- your knowledge and skills in relation to any particular role or responsibility of your current post.

The extent of expertise you should possess will depend on your level of responsibility for a particular function or task. You may be personally responsible for that function or task, or you may contribute or delegate responsibility for it. Your learning needs should take into account your aspirations for the future too – personal or career development for you, or improvements in the way you deliver care in your practice. Look at Chapter 2 for more ideas on how you will identify your learning or service development needs.

Group and summarise your service development needs from the exercises you have carried out. Grade them according to the priority you set. You may put one at a higher priority because it fits in with service development needs established in the business plan of the trust or practice, or put another lower because it does not fit in with other activities that your organisation has in their current development plan for the next 12 months. If you have identified a service development need by several different methods of assessment or with several different patient groups or clinical conditions, then it will have a higher priority than something only identified once. Notify the service development needs you have identified to those responsible for agreeing and implementing the development plans of the trust and/or practice.

Look back at your aspirations and standards set out in Stages 1 and 2. Match your learning or service development needs with one or more of these standards, or others that you have set yourself.

Stage 4: Make and carry out a learning and action plan with a timetable for your personal and service development

If you have not identified any learning needs for yourself or the service as a whole, you should omit Stage 4 and tidy up the presentation of your evidence for inclusion in your portfolio as at the end of Stage 5.

Think about whether:

- you have defined your learning objectives – what you need to learn to be able to attain the standards and outcomes you have described in Stage 2
- you can justify spending time and effort on the topics you prioritised in Stage 3. Is the topic important enough to your work, the NHS as a whole or patient safety? Does the clinical or non-clinical event occur sufficiently often to warrant the time spent?
- the time and resources for learning about that topic or making the associated changes to service delivery are available. Check that you are not trying to do too much too quickly, or you will become discouraged
- learning about that topic will make a difference to the care you or others can provide for patients
- and how one topic fits in with other topics you have identified to learn more about. Have you achieved a good balance across your areas of work or between your personal aspirations and the basic requirements of the service?

Decide on what method of learning is most appropriate for your task or role or the standards you are expecting to attain or sustain. You may have already identified your preferred learning style – but read up on this elsewhere if you are unsure.[7]

Describe how you will carry out your learning tasks and what you will do by a specified time. State how your learning will be applied and how and when it will be evaluated. Build in some staging posts so that you do not suddenly get to the end of 12 months and discover that you have only done half of your plan.

Your action plan should also include your role in remedying any gaps in service delivery that you identified in Stage 3 that are within the remit of your responsibility.

Stage 5: Document your learning, competence, performance and standards of service delivery

You might choose to document that you have attained your defined outcomes by repeating the learning needs assessment that you started with. You could record your increased confidence and competence in dealing with situations that you previously avoided or performed inadequately.

You might incorporate your assessment of what has been gained in a study of another area that overlaps.

Preparing your portfolio[8-10]

Use your portfolio of evidence of what you have learnt and your standards of practice to:

- identify significant experiences to serve as important sources of learning
- reflect on the learning that arose from those experiences
- demonstrate learning in practice
- analyse and identify further learning needs and ways in which these needs can be met.

Your documentation might include all sorts of things, not just formal audits – although they make a good start. It might include reports of educational activities attended, statements of your roles and responsibilities, copies of publications you have read and critically appraised, and reports of your work. You could incorporate observations by others, evaluations of yourself observing other colleagues and how their practice differs from yours, descriptions of self-improvements, a video of typical activity, materials that demonstrate your skills to others, products of your input or learning – a new protocol for example. Box 1.3 gives a list of material you might include in your portfolio.

Box 1.3:   Possible contents of a portfolio
- Workload logs
- Case descriptions
- Videos
- Audiotapes
- Patient satisfaction surveys
- Research surveys
- Report of change or innovation
- Commentaries on published literature or books
- Records of critical incidents and learning points
- Notes from formal teaching sessions with reference to clinical work or other evidence

---

Once you are preparing to submit the portfolio for a discussion with a colleague (for example, at an appraisal) or assessment (for example, for a university postgraduate award or revalidation), write a self-assessment of your previous action plan. You might integrate your self-assessment into your PDP to show what you have achieved and what gaps you have still to address. Decide where are you now and where you want to be in one, three or five years' time. Select items from your portfolio for inclusion for each part of the documentation – you might have one compartment of your portfolio per specialty topic or section heading from *Good Medical Practice*.[3]

Make sure all references are included and the documentation in your portfolio is as accurate and complete as possible. Organise how you have shown your learning steps and your standards of practice so that it is indexed and cross-referenced to the relevant sections of the paperwork. Discuss the contents of your portfolio with a colleague or a mentor to gain other people's perspectives of your work and look for blind spots.

Include evidence of your competence as a GP with a special interest (GPwSI)

You may have a particular expertise or special interest in a clinical field or non-clinical area such as management, teaching or research. It may be that you have a lead role or responsibility in your practice for chronic disease management of clinical conditions such as diabetes, asthma, mental health or coronary heart disease. Or you may be employed by a PCO or hospital trust as a GPwSI to:

- lead in the development of services

- deliver a procedure-based service
- deliver an opinion-based service.

There is little consistency in extent of training or qualifications at present within or across the various GPwSI specialty areas.[11] Look at Chapter 4 for an example of what is expected in drug misuse. Whatever your role or responsibility or expertise, your portfolio should include examples of evidence that show that you are competent, and that you have a consistently good performance in your specialty area. You may have parallel appraisals that you can include from your employer – for example, the university if you have a research or teaching post, or a hospital consultant if he or she supervises you in the clinical specialty.

When you gather evidence of your performance at work, try to document as many aspects of your work at one time as you can, so that for example an audit covers as many of the key headings from *Good Medical Practice* (*see* Box 1.1 page 5) as possible.[3] When you are identifying what you need to learn, or gaps in service delivery, make sure that you involve patients and show how you interact with the team. This gives you evidence about 'relationships with patients' and 'working with colleagues' as well as the clinical area you are focusing on or auditing.

Link your cycles of evidence to service developments rewarded by the General Medical Services (GMS) Contract or Personal Medical Services (PMS) arrangements

The areas within the quality framework will probably be the ones that you prioritise in your PDP when looking at your service development needs.[12] The four main components of the quality framework are all relevant to your personal and professional development. The clinical and organisational standards may be those which you are aiming for in Stage 2 of the evidence cycle (*see* Figure 1.1). Achieving the standards in the quality framework will follow on from the descriptions of an excellent GP (Stage 1). Identifying personal learning needs and service development needs, that is, the gaps between baseline and specified standards in the quality framework, are in Stage 3. Making and carrying out your personal learning plan and service improvements in line with patients' experience is in Stage 4. Producing the documentation that shows you have attained the clinical or organisational standards required for core or additional services and responded to patients' views is in Stage 5.

References

1   Wakley G, Chambers R and Field S (2000) *Continuing Professional Development in Primary Care.* Radcliffe Medical Press, Oxford.

2   Royal College of General Practitioners/General Practitioners Committee (2002) *Good Medical Practice for General Practitioners.* Royal College of General Practitioners, London.

3   General Medical Council (2001) *Good Medical Practice.* General Medical Council, London.

4   Department of Health (1998) *A First Class Service.* Department of Health, London.

5   Department of Health (1999) *Supporting Doctors, Protecting Patients.* Department of Health, London.

6   General Medical Council (2003) *Licence to Practise and Revalidation for Doctors.* General Medical Council, London. www.revalidationuk.info

7   Mohanna K, Wall D and Chambers R (2003) *Teaching Made Easy: a manual for health professionals* (2e). Radcliffe Medical Press, Oxford.

8   Royal College of General Practitioners (1993) *Portfolio-based Learning in General Practice.* Occasional Paper 63, Royal College of General Practitioners, London.

9   Challis M (1999) AMEE Medical education guide No 11 (revised): portfolio-based learning and assessment in medical education. *Medical Teacher.* **21(4):** 370–86.

10 Chambers C, Wakley G, Field S and Ellis S (2003) *Appraisal for the Apprehensive.* Radcliffe Medical Press, Oxford.

11 www.gpwsi.org

12 General Practitioners Committee/NHS Confederation (2003) *New GMS Contract. Investing in general practice.* General Practitioners Committee/NHS Confederation, London.

2

Practical ways to identify your learning and service needs as part of the documentation of your competence and performance

Setting standards to show that you are competent

> Doctors 'must be committed to lifelong learning and be responsible for maintaining the medical knowledge and clinical and team skills necessary for the provision of quality care.'[1]

You could make a good start by describing your roles and responsibilities. This will help you to define what your competence should be now, or what competence you are hoping to attain (for instance as a GPwSI). Once you have your definition, you can recognise whether you have, or lack in some part, the necessary competence. If there are no accepted descriptions of competence in the area you are focusing on, then you will have to start from scratch. You might compile your description from national guidelines such as in the National Service Frameworks or health strategies. Usually you can find guidance about competency from specialist sources such as primary care associations for clinical topics or the various Royal Colleges. The Department of Health in England has worked with the Royal College of General Practitioners (RCGP) to describe the competency of GPs with special clinical interests in many clinical areas.[2]

A good definition of competence is someone who is: 'able to perform the tasks and roles required to the expected standard'.[3]

You will need to describe the standards expected in the range of tasks and roles you undertake and reference the source of standard setting. If professionals, or their organisations, are the only people involved in setting those standards, consider whether you should amend or extend the standards, tasks or roles by considering other perspectives such as those of patients or the NHS as a whole.

There is a difference between being competent, and performing in a consistently competent manner. You need to be motivated to perform consistently well and enabled to do so with efficient systems and sufficient resources. You will require sufficient numbers of other competent doctors or staff and available infrastructure such as diagnostic and treatment resources.[4]

Choose methods in Stage 3 (*see* Chapter 1) to demonstrate your standards of performance and identify any learning needs that span different topic areas, to reduce duplication and maximise the usefulness of your learning. Collecting evidence of more than one aspect of your competence or performance cuts down the overall amount of work underpinning your PDP or included in your appraisal portfolio.

Use several methods to identify your learning needs and/or gaps in your service development or delivery, so that you validate the findings of one method by another. No one method will give you reliable information about the gaps in your knowledge, skills or attitudes or everyday service. Does what you think about your performance match with what others in the team or patients think of how you practise in your everyday work? It is particularly difficult to determine what it is you 'don't know you don't know' by yourself, yet it is vital that you identify and rectify those gaps. Other people may be able to tell you what you need to learn quite readily. Colleagues from different disciplines could usefully comment on any shortfalls in how your work interfaces with theirs.

Patients or people who don't use your services could tell you whether the way you operate or provide services is off-putting or inappropriate. There may be data about your performance or that of your practice that could point out those gaps in your knowledge or skills of which you were previously unaware.

Determine what it is that you 'don't know you don't know' by:

- asking patients, users and non-users of your service
- comparing your performance against best practice or that of peers
- comparing your performance against objectives in business plans or national directives
- asking colleagues from different disciplines about shortfalls in how your work interfaces with theirs.

Identify your learning needs – how you can find out if you need to be better at doing your job

You may decide to use a few selected methods to gather baseline evidence of your performance, focused on your specific area of expertise. You may target other topics or areas at the same time that are relevant to the various sections of the GMC's booklet *Good Medical Practice*.[5] For this type of combined assessment, you might use several of the methods described in this chapter such as:

- constructive feedback from peers or patients
- 360° feedback
- self-assessment, or review by others, using a rating scale to assess your skills and attitudes
- comparison with protocols and guidelines for checking how well procedures are followed
- audit: various types and applications
- significant event audit
- eliciting patient views such as satisfaction surveys
- a SWOT (strengths, weaknesses, opportunities and threats) or SCOT (strengths, challenges, opportunities and threats) analysis
- reading and reflecting
- educational review.

Several of these methods will also be useful for identifying service development needs – you can look at the gaps identified from both the personal and service perspectives at the same time using the same method.

Seek feedback

Find colleagues who will give you constructive feedback about your performance and practice. The golden rule for giving constructive feedback is to give positive praise of things that have been well done first. Sometimes colleagues launch straight in to criticise faults when asked for their views. The Pendleton model of the giving of feedback is widely used in the health setting (*see* Box 2.1).[6]

Box 2.1: The Pendleton model of giving feedback

1 The 'learner' goes first and performs the activity.
2 Questions from the teacher clarify any facts.
3 The 'learner' says what they thought was done well.

4 The 'teacher' says what they thought was done well.
5 The 'learner' says what could be improved upon.
6 The 'teacher' says what could be improved upon.
7 Both discuss ideas for improvements in a helpful and constructive manner.

360° feedback

This collects together perceptions from a number of different participants as shown in Figure 2.1.

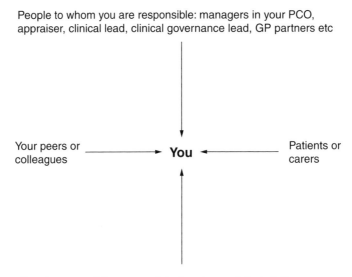

Figure 2.1:   360° feedback.

The wider the spread of people giving feedback, the more rounded the picture. Each individual gives a feedback questionnaire to at least three people in each of the groups above. An independent person then collects and collates the questionnaires and discusses the results with the individual. Computerised versions are available from commercial companies.[7] The main disadvantage of this method is that it can sometimes be spoilt by malicious comments against which individuals cannot readily defend themselves.

Self-assess or gain another person's perspective on your standard of practice or service delivery

You might describe any aspect of your practice as statements (A to G as in Box 2.2) about your competence or performance for you to self-assess or others to give you feedback or comments by marking the extent to which they agree on the linear scales below. You could use the descriptions of an excellent GP in *Good Medical Practice for General Practitioners*[8] as we have done in relating statements in Box 2.2 to consultation skills. For instance, if statement A is: 'I consistently treat patients politely and with consideration',[8] you could self-assess the extent to which you agree. Alternatively, you could ask colleagues or patients to fill in the assessment form. Objective feedback from external assessment is usually more reliable than your own self-assessment when you may have blind spots about your own performance. As you become more confident in this method of reviewing your competence, you might emphasise how consistent you are in your application of good practice – so in the statements below we have sometimes included 'consistently', 'always' or 'usually'. You can set your own challenges. If you have a mentor or a 'buddy' in the practice with whom you learn, you might discuss and reflect on the completed marking grids with him or her.

Box 2.2:   Marking grid: circle the number which represents your views or feelings about each statement – complete the grid on more than one occasion and compare results over time

A   I consistently treat patients politely and with consideration.

STRONGLY AGREE   to   STRONGLY DISAGREE

1----------------2----------------3----------------4----------------5----------------6

B   I am aware of how my personal beliefs could affect the care offered to the patient, and take care not to impose my own beliefs and values.

STRONGLY AGREE   to   STRONGLY DISAGREE

1----------------2----------------3----------------4----------------5----------------6

C   I always treat all patients equally and ensure that some groups are not favoured at the expense of others.

STRONGLY AGREE   to   STRONGLY DISAGREE

1----------------2----------------3----------------4----------------5----------------6

D   I try to maintain a relationship with the patient or family when a mistake has occurred.

STRONGLY AGREE   to   STRONGLY DISAGREE

1----------------2----------------3----------------4----------------5----------------6

E   I always obtain informed consent to treatment.

STRONGLY AGREE   to   STRONGLY DISAGREE

1----------------2----------------3----------------4----------------5----------------6

F   I usually involve patients in decisions about their care.

STRONGLY AGREE   to   STRONGLY DISAGREE

1----------------2----------------3----------------4----------------5----------------6

G   I always respect the right of patients to refuse treatments or tests.

STRONGLY AGREE   to   STRONGLY DISAGREE

1----------------2----------------3----------------4----------------5----------------6

Compare your performance against protocols or guidelines

Are you familiar with all the protocols or guidelines that are used by someone, somewhere in the practice? You might determine your learning needs and those of other practice team members by piling all the protocols or guidelines that exist in your practice in a big heap and rationalising them so that you have a common set across the practice. Working as a team you can compare your own knowledge and usual practice with others and with protocols or guidelines recommended by the National Institute for Clinical Excellence (NICE)[9] or National Service Frameworks or the Scottish Intercollegiate Guidelines Network (SIGN).[10]

Alternatively, you might compare your own practice against a protocol or guideline that is generally accepted at a national or local level. You could audit the standard of your practice to find out how often you adhere to such a protocol or guideline, and if you can justify why you deviate from the recommendations.

Audit

Audit is:

the method used by health professionals to assess, evaluate, and improve the care of patients in a systematic way, to enhance their health and quality of life.[11]

The five steps of the audit cycle are shown in Box 2.3.

Box 2.3: The five steps of the audit cycle

1 Describe the criteria and standards you are trying to achieve.
2 Measure your current performance of how well you are providing care or services in an objective way.
3 Compare your performance against criteria and standards.
4 Identify the need for change – to performance, adjustment of criteria or standards, resources, available data.
5 Make any required changes as necessary and re-audit later.

Performance or practice is often broken down for the purposes of audit into the three aspects of structure, process and outcome. Structural audits might concern resources such as equipment, premises, skills, people, etc. Process audits focus on what is done to the patient: for instance, clinical protocols and guidelines. Audits of outcomes consider the impact of care or services on the patient and might include patient satisfaction, health gains and effectiveness of care or services. You might look at aspects of quality of the structure, process and outcome of the delivery of any clinical field – focusing on access, equity of care between different groups in the population, efficiency, economy, effectiveness for individual patients, etc.[11]

Set standards for your performance, find out how you are doing, search to find out best practice, make the changes and then re-audit the care given to patients in the future with the same problem. Some variations on audit include:

- *Case note analysis.* This gives an insight into your current practice. It might be a retrospective review of a random selection of notes, or a prospective survey of consecutive patients with the same condition as they present to see you.
- *Peer review.* Compare an area of practice with other individual professionals or managers; or compare practice teams as a whole. An independent body might compare all practices in one area e.g. within a primary care trust (PCT) or organisation so that like is compared with like. Feedback may be arranged to protect participants' identities so that only the individual person or practice knows their own identity, the rest being anonymised, for example by giving each practice a number. Where there is mutual trust and an open learning culture, peer review does not need to be anonymised and everyone can learn together about making improvements in practice.
- *Criteria-based audit.* This compares clinical practice with specific standards, guidelines or protocols. Re-audit of changes should demonstrate improvements in the quality of patient care.
- *External audit.* Prescribing advisors or managers in PCOs can supply information about indicators of performance for audit. Visits from external

bodies such as the Healthcare Commission expose the PCO or hospital trust in England and Wales to external audit.

- *Tracer criteria*. Assessing the quality of care of a 'tracer' condition may be used to represent the quality of care of other similar conditions or more complex problems. Tracer criteria should be easily defined and measured. For instance, if you were to audit the extent to which you reviewed repeat prescriptions, you might focus on a drug such as levothyroxine and generalise from your audit results to your likely performance with other medications.

Significant event audit

Think of an incident where a patient or you experienced an adverse event. This might be an unexpected death, an unplanned pregnancy, an avoidable side-effect from prescribed medication, a violent attack on a member of staff, or an angry outburst in public by you or a work colleague. You can review the case and reflect on the sequence of events that led to that critical event occurring. It is likely that there were a multitude of factors leading up to that significant event. You should take the case to a multidisciplinary meeting to reflect and analyse what were the triggers, causes and consequences of the event. Complete the significant event audit cycle by planning what individuals or the practice as a whole might do to avoid a similar event happening in future. This might include undertaking further learning and/or making appropriate changes to the practice or your systems.

The steps of a significant event audit are shown in Box 2.4.

Box 2.4:   Steps of a significant event audit

- *Step 1*: Describe who was involved, what time of day, what the task/activity was, the context and any other relevant information.
- *Step 2*: Reflect on the effects of the event on the participants and the professionals involved.
- *Step 3*: Discuss the reasons for the event or situation arising with other colleagues, review case notes or other records.
- *Step 4*: Decide how you or others might have behaved differently. Describe your options for how the procedures at work might be changed to minimise or eliminate the chances of the event recurring.
- *Step 5*: Plan changes that are needed, how they will be implemented, who will be responsible for what and when, what further training or resources are required. Then carry out the changes.
- *Step 6*: Re-audit later to see whether changes to procedures or new knowledge and skills are having the desired effects. Give feedback to the practice team.

An assessment by an external body

This is a traditional way of showing that you are competent by taking and passing an examination. It is a good way of testing recalled knowledge in a written or oral examination, or establishing how you behave in a clinical situation on the day of a practical examination, but not much good for measuring anything else. A summative examination (i.e. done at the end of a course of study) gives a measure of your learning up to that date.

You might undertake an objective test of your knowledge and skills. Examples are a computer-based test in the form of multiple choice questions and patient management problems as in the RCGP's phased evaluation programme (PEP) CD-ROMs (email pep@rcgp-scotland.org.uk) or the Apollo programme available from BMJ Publishing.[12] Various other organisations give multiple choice questionnaires that you can complete on paper and record in your portfolio.[13,14]

Elicit the views of patients

Part of meeting the criteria for relationships with patients in *Good Medical Practice*[5] might be to assess patients' satisfaction with:

- you
- your practice
- the local hospital's way of working
- other services available in your locality.

Avoid surveys where questions are relatively superficial or biased. A more specific enquiry should uncover particular elements of patients' dissatisfaction, which will be more useful if you are trying to identify your learning needs. Use a well-validated patient questionnaire, instead of risking producing your own version with ambiguities and flaws, such as the General Practice Assessment Questionnaire (GPAQ)[15] or the Doctors' Interpersonal Skills Questionnaire (DISQ).[16] Many doctors and practice teams have used these patient survey methods, providing a bank of data against which to compare your performance.

Other sources of feedback from patients might be obtained through suggestion boxes for patients to contribute comments, or the practice team recording all patients' suggestions and complaints however trivial, looking for patterns in the comments received.

There will be learning to be had from every complaint – even if the complaint does not have any substance, there should be something to learn about the shortfall in communication between you and the complainant.

The evolution of the 'expert patient programme' should mean that there is a pool of well informed patients with chronic conditions who can contribute their insights into what you (or the service) need to learn from a patient's perspective.[17]

Strengths, weaknesses (or challenges), opportunities and threats (SWOT or SCOT) analysis

You can undertake a SWOT (or SCOT) analysis of your own performance or that of your practice team or practice organisation, working it out on your own, or with a workmate or mentor, or with a group of colleagues. Brainstorm the strengths, weaknesses (or challenges), opportunities and threats of your role or circumstances.

Strengths and weaknesses (or challenges) of your roles might relate to your clinical knowledge or skills, experience, expertise, decision making, communication skills, interprofessional relationships, political skills, timekeeping, organisational skills, teaching skills, or research skills. Strengths and weaknesses (or challenges) of the practice organisation might relate to most of these aspects as well as the way resources are allocated, overall efficiency and the degree to which the practice is patient centred.

Opportunities might relate to your unexploited experience or potential strengths, expected changes in the NHS, or resources for which you might bid. For example, you might train for and set up a special interest post.

Threats will include factors and circumstances that prevent you from achieving your aims for personal, professional and practice development or service improvements. They might be to do with your health, turnover in the practice team, or time-limited investment by the PCO.

List the important factors in your SWOT (or SCOT) analysis in order of priority, through discussion with colleagues and independent people from outside your practice. Draw up goals and a timed action plan for you or the practice team to follow.

Informal conversations – in the corridor, over coffee

You learn such a lot when chatting with colleagues at coffee time or over a meal and can become aware of your learning or service development needs at these times. This is when you realise that other people are doing things differently from you, and if they seem to be doing it better and achieving more, you can challenge yourself to decide if this matter could be one of your blind spots. Note down your thoughts before you forget them so that you can reflect on them later.

Online discussion groups may provide another source of informal exchanges with colleagues. If you find this difficult to start with, you might 'lurk', viewing the comments and views of other people until you feel confident enough to contribute. Record any observations that you find useful and reflect on how they might inform your own practice.

Observe your work environment and role

Observation could be informal and opportunistic, or more systematic working through a structured checklist. One method of self-assessment might be to audiotape yourself at work dealing with patients (after obtaining patients' informed consent). Listen to the tape afterwards to appraise your communication and consultation skills – on your own or with a friend or colleague. If you have access to video equipment, you might use this instead.

Look at the equipment in your practice or your emergency bag. Do you know how to operate it properly? Assess yourself undertaking practical procedures or ask someone to watch you operate the equipment or undertaking the practical procedure and give you feedback about your performance.

Analyse the various roles and responsibilities of your current posts. Compare your level of expertise against national standards such as in the Knowledge and Skills Framework for England from the Department of Health or a job evaluation framework as part of the Agenda for Change initiative.[18,19] Determine if you can meet the requirements, or, if not, what deficiencies need to be made good.

You might combine one of the methods of identifying your learning needs already described such as an audit or SWOT analysis and apply it to 'observing your work environment or role', describing your relationship with other members of the multidisciplinary team for example, or reviewing how their roles and responsibilities interface with yours.

Read and reflect

When reading articles in respected journals, reflect on what the key messages mean for you in your situation. Note down topics about which you know little but that are relevant to your work, and calculate if you have further learning needs not met by the article you are reading. If the article is relevant to your practice, record what changes you will make and how you will make the changes. Record how you will impart your new knowledge to others in your practice.

Educational review

You might find a buddy or work colleague, CPD tutor, or a clinical tutor or clinical supervisor with whom you can have an informal or formal discussion about your performance, job situation and learning needs. You might draw up a learning contract as a result with a timed plan of action.

Identify your service needs – how you can find out if there are gaps in services or how you deliver care

Now focus your attention on the needs of your practice or the PCO. The standards of service delivery should be those that allow you to practise as a competent clinician. You may be competent but be unable to perform or practise to a competent level if the resources available to you are inadequate, or other colleagues have insufficient knowledge or skills to support you. You cannot be expected to take responsibility for ensuring that resources you need to be able to practise in a competent manner are available. However, as a professional you should play a significant role in collecting evidence to make a case for the need for essential resources to your GP colleagues, the practice manager, staff at the trust or PCO or whoever is appropriate.

Some of the methods you might use are described below and include:

- involving patients and the public in giving you feedback about the quality and quantity of your services
- monitoring access and availability to care
- undertaking a force-field analysis
- assessing risk
- evaluating the standards of care or services you provide
- comparing the systems in your practice with those required by legislation
- considering your patient population's health needs
- reviewing teamwork
- assessing the quality of your services
- reflecting on whether you are providing cost-effective care and services.

Involve patients and the public in giving you feedback about the quality and quantity of your services

Patient and public involvement may occur at three levels:

1 for individual patients about their own care
2 for patients and the public about the range and quality of health services on offer
3 in planning and organising health service developments.

The phrase 'patient and public involvement' is used here to mean individual involvement as a user, patient or carer, or public involvement that includes the processes of consultation and participation.[20]

   If a patient involvement or public consultation exercise is to be meaningful, it has to involve people who represent the section of the population that the exercise is about. You will have to set up systems to actively seek out and involve people from minority groups or those with sensory impairments such as blind and deaf people.

   Before you start:

- define the purpose
- be realistic about the magnitude of the planned exercise
- select an appropriate method or several methods depending on the target population and your resources
- obtain the commitment of everyone who will be affected by the exercise
- frame the method in accordance with your perspective
- write the protocol.

You might hold focus groups, or set up a patient panel, or invite feedback and help from a patient participation group. You could interview patients selected either at random from the patient population or for their experience of a particular condition or circumstance.

Monitor access to and availability of healthcare

Access and availability

You could look at waiting times to see a health professional by using:

- computerised appointment lists or paper and pen to record the time of arrival, the time of the appointment, the time seen
- the next available appointments that can easily be monitored by computer, or more painfully by manual searches of the appointment books.

Compare the results at intervals (a spreadsheet is a good way to do this). Do you or your staff have learning needs in relation to the use of technology, or new ways of redesigning the service you offer?

Referrals to other agencies and hospitals

You might audit and re-audit the time taken from the date the patient is seen to:

*   the referral being sent (do you need more secretarial time?)
*   the date the patient is seen by the other agency (could the patient be seen elsewhere quicker or do you need to liaise with other agencies over referrals?)
*   the date the patient's needs have been met by investigation, diagnosis, treatment, provision of aid or support, etc (can you influence how quickly these are completed?).

Identify any learning needs here. For instance, new methods of teamwork with a different mix of skills between doctors, nurses and non-clinically qualified assistants could provide extra services in the practice, or you, or a colleague, might retrain to become a GP with a special clinical interest.

Draw up a force-field analysis

This tool will help you to identify and focus down on the positive and negative forces in your work and to gain an overview of the weighting of these factors. Draw a horizontal or vertical line in the middle of a sheet of paper. Label one side 'positive' and the other side 'negative'. Draw bars to represent individual positive drivers that motivate you on one side of the line, and factors that are demotivating on the other negative side of the line. The thickness and length of the bars should represent the extent of the influence; that is, a short, narrow bar will indicate that the positive or negative factor has a minor influence and a long, wide bar a major effect. *See* Box 2.5 for an example.

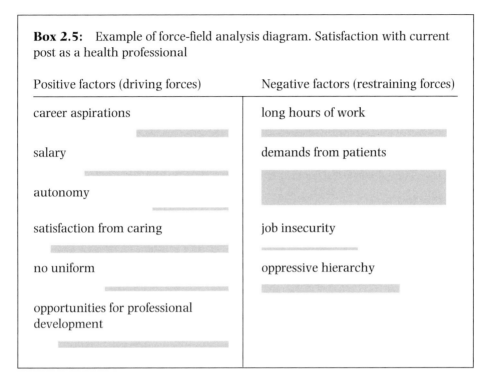

Box 2.5:   Example of force-field analysis diagram. Satisfaction with current post as a health professional

Positive factors (driving forces)	Negative factors (restraining forces)
career aspirations	long hours of work
salary	demands from patients
autonomy	
satisfaction from caring	job insecurity
no uniform	oppressive hierarchy
opportunities for professional development	

Take an overview of the resulting force-field diagram and consider if you are content with things as they are, or can think of ways to boost the positive side and minimise the negative factors. You can do this part of the exercise on your own, with a peer or a small group in the practice, or with a mentor or someone from outside the practice. The exercise should help you to realise the extent to which a known influence in your life, or in the practice as a whole, is a positive or negative factor. Make a personal or organisational action plan to create the situations and opportunities to boost the positive factors in your life and minimise the bars on the negative side.

Assess risk

Risk assessment might entail evaluating the risks to the health or wellbeing or competence of yourself, staff and/or patients in your practice or workplace, and deciding on the action needed to minimise or eliminate those risks.[21]

- *A hazard*: something with the potential to cause harm.
- *A risk*: the likelihood of that potential to cause harm being realised.

There are five steps to risk assessment:

1 look for and list the hazards
2 decide who might be harmed and how
3 evaluate the risks arising from the hazards and decide whether existing precautions are adequate or more should be done
4 record the findings
5 review your assessment from time to time and revise it if necessary.

You do not want to spend a lot of time and effort identifying risks or making changes if they do not matter much. When you have identified a risk, consider:

• is the risk large?
• does it happen often?
• is it a significant risk?

Risks may be prevented, avoided, minimised or managed where they cannot be eliminated. You, your colleagues and your staff may need to learn how to do this.

Record significant events where someone has experienced an adverse event or had a near miss – as part of you identifying your service development needs on an ongoing basis. Most significant incidents do not have one cause. Usually there are faults in the system, which are compounded by someone or several people being careless, tired, overworked or ill-informed. Cultivate an atmosphere of openness and discussion without blame so that you can all learn from the significant event. If people think they will be blamed they will hide the incident and no one will be able to prevent it happening again. Look for *all* the causes and try to remedy as many as possible to prevent the situation from arising in the future.

Evaluate the standards of services or care you provide

Keep your evaluation as simple as possible. Avoid wasting resources on unnecessarily bureaucratic evaluation. Design the evaluation so that you:

• specify the event (such as a service) to be evaluated – define broad issues, set priorities against strategic goals, time and resources, seek agreement on the nature and scope of the task
• describe the expected impact of the programme or activity and who will be affected
• define the criteria of success – these might relate to structure, process or outcome
• identify the information required to demonstrate the achievements of the programme or activity. The record might include: observing behaviour;

data from existing records; prospective recording by the subjects of the programme or by the recipients and staff of the activity
- determine the time frame for the evaluation
- specify who collects the data for all stages in the delivery of the programme or activity, and the respective deadlines
- review and refine the objectives of the programme or activity and check that they are appropriate for the outcomes and impact you expect.

What to evaluate?

You could:

- adopt any, or all, of the six aspects of the health service's performance assessment framework (*see* Box 2.6)
- agree milestones and goals at stages in your programme or adopt others such as those relating to the National Service Frameworks for coronary heart disease or mental health
- evaluate the extent to which you achieve the outcome(s) starting with an objective. Alternatively, you might evaluate how conducive is the context of the programme, or activity, to achieving the anticipated outcomes
- undertake regular audits of aspects of the structure, process and outcome of a service or project to see if you have achieved what you expected when you established the criteria and standards of the audit programme
- evaluate the various components of a new system or programme: the activities, personnel involved, provision of services, organisational structure, precise goals and interventions.

Box 2.6:   The six aspects of the NHS performance assessment framework

1 Health improvement
2 Fair access
3 Effective delivery
4 Efficiency
5 Patient/carer experience
6 Health outcomes

Computer search

The extent to which you can evaluate your practice will depend on the quality of your records and the extent to which you use the capacity of your practice computer. Compare the results of a computerised search for all those using one type of treatment with another. Make appropriate changes to your systems depending on what the computer search reveals. Put your plan into action and monitor with repeat searches at regular intervals.

Look at your learning or service development needs by analysing data from practice records to:

- look at trends and patterns of illness
- devise and use clinical guidelines and decision support systems as part of evidence-based practice
- audit what you are doing
- provide the information on which to base decisions on commissioning and management
- support epidemiology, research and teaching activities.

Compare the systems in your practice with those required by legislation

Legislation changes quite frequently. As an employer, a GP needs to keep abreast of the legislation or ensure that the practice manager does so. You could start by comparing the systems in your practice with those required by the Disability Discrimination Act (1995) and health and safety legislation.

Consider your patient population's health needs

Create a detailed profile of your practice population. Ask your PCO or public health lead for information about your practice population and comparative information about the general population living in the district – morbidity and mortality statistics, referral patterns, age/sex mix, ethnicity, and population trends.

Include information about the wider determinants of health such as housing, numbers of the population in, and types of, employment, geographical location, the environment, crime and safety, educational attainment and socio-economic data. Make a note of any particular health problems such as higher than average teenage pregnancy rates or drug misuse. Focus on the current state of health inequalities within your practice population or between your practice population and the district as a whole. It may be that circumstances change, which in turn alters the proportion of minority groups in your practice population – such as if a continuing care home opens up in your practice area, or there is an influx of homeless people or asylum seekers into your locality.

Review teamwork

You can measure how effective the team is[22] – evaluate whether the team has:

- clear goals and objectives
- accountability and authority
- individual roles for members
- shared tasks
- regular internal formal and informal communication
- full participation by members
- confrontation of conflict
- feedback to individuals
- feedback about team performance
- outside recognition
- two-way external communication
- team rewards.

Assess the quality of your services

Quality may be subdivided into eight components: equity, access, acceptability and responsiveness, appropriateness, communication, continuity, effectiveness and efficiency.[23]

You might use the matrix in Box 2.7 as a way of ordering your approach to auditing a particular topic with the eight aspects of quality on the vertical axis and structure, process and outcome on the horizontal axis.[24] In this way you can generate up to 24 aspects of a particular topic. You might then focus on several aspects to look at the quality of patient care or services from various angles.

Box 2.7:   Matrix for assessing the quality of a clinical service

You might look at the structure, process or outcome of communicating test results to patients, for example.

	Structure	Process	Outcome
Equity			
Access			
Acceptability and responsiveness			
Appropriateness			
Communication	Hospital report	Feedback	Action taken
Continuity			
Effectiveness			
Efficiency			

Look for service development needs reflecting why patients receive a poor quality of service such as:

- inadequately trained staff or staff with poor levels of competence
- lack of confidentiality
- staff not being trained in the management of emergency situations
- doctors or nurses not being contactable in an emergency or being ineffective
- treatment being unavailable due to poor management of resources or services
- poor management of the arrangements for home visiting
- insufficient numbers of available staff for the workload
- qualifications of locums or deputising staff being unknown or inadequate for the posts they are filling
- arrangements for transfer of information from one team member to another being inadequate
- team members not acting on information received.

Many of these items will need action as a team, but for some of them, it may be your responsibility to ensure that adequate standards are met.

Reflect on whether you are providing cost-effective care and services

Cost-effectiveness is not synonymous with 'cheap'. A cost-effective inter-vention is one which gives a better or equivalent benefit from the intervention in question for lower or equivalent cost, or where the relative improvement in outcome is higher than the relative difference in cost. In other words being cost-effective means having the best outcomes for the least input. Using the term 'cost-effective' implies that you have considered potential alternatives.

An intervention must first be considered *clinically* effective to warrant investigation into its potential to be *cost*-effective. Evidence-based practice must incorporate clinical judgement. You have to interpret the evidence when it comes to applying it to individual patients, whether it is evidence about clinical effectiveness or cost-effectiveness. A new or alternative treatment or intervention should be compared directly with the previous best treatment or intervention.

An economic evaluation is a comparative analysis of two or more alterna-tives in terms of their costs and consequences. There are four different types as shown in Box 2.8.

Box 2.8: The four types of economic evaluation

1 *Cost-effectiveness analysis* is used to compare the effectiveness of two interventions with the same treatment objectives.
2 *Cost minimisation* compares the costs of alternative treatments that have identical health outcomes.
3 *Cost–utility analysis* enables the effects of alternative interventions to be measured against a combination of life expectancy and quality of life; common outcome measures are quality adjusted life years (QALYs) or health-related quality of life (hrqol).
4 *Cost–benefit analysis* is a technique designed to determine the feasibility of a project, plan, management or treatment by quantifying its costs and benefits. It is often difficult to determine these accurately in relation to health.

While health valuation is unavoidable, it cannot be objective. You will probably have learning needs around what subjective method is best to use.[25]

Efficiency is sometimes confused with effectiveness. Being efficient means obtaining the most quality from the least expenditure, or the required level of quality for the least expenditure. To measure efficiency you need to make a judgement about the level of quality of the 'purchase' and be able to relate it to 'price'. 'Price' alone does not measure efficiency. Quality is the indicator used in combination with price to assess if something is more efficient. So, cost-effectiveness is a measure of efficiency and suggests that costs have been related to effectiveness.

Consider whether you have service development needs. Discuss whether:

- the current skill mix in your team is appropriate
- more cost-effective alternative types of delivery of care are available
- sufficient staff training exists for those taking on new roles and responsibilities.

Set priorities: how you match what's needed with what's possible

You and your colleagues will have been able to make a wish list after following the previous Stages 3A and 3B undertaking a variety of needs assessments. Group and summarise your learning and service development needs from the exercises you have carried out. Grade them according to the priority you set. You may put one at a higher priority because it fits in with learning needs established from another section, or put another lower because it does not fit in with other activities that you will put into your learning plan for the next

12 months. If you have identified a learning need by several different methods of assessment, then it will have a higher priority than something only identified once in your PDP. Collect information from all the team, the patients, users and carers to feed back before you make a decision on how to progress. Remember to consider external influences such as the National Service Frameworks, NICE guidance, governmental priorities, priorities of your PCO, the content of the Local Delivery Plan, etc.

Select those topics that are tied into organisational priorities, have clear aims and objectives and are achievable within your time and resource constraints. When ranking topics for learning or action in order of priority (Stage 4) consider whether:

- the project aims and objectives are clearly defined
- the topic is important:
  - for the population served (e.g. the size of the problem and/or its severity)
  - for the skills, knowledge or attitudes of the individual or team
- it is feasible
- it is affordable
- it will make enough difference
- it fits in with other priorities.

You will still have more ideas than can possibly be implemented. Remember the highest priority – the health service is for patients that use it or who will do so in the future.

References

1 Medical Professionalism Project (2002) Medical professionalism in the new millennium: a physicians' charter. *Lancet.* **359:** 520–2.

2 www.gpwsi.org

3 Eraut M and du Boulay B (2000) *Developing the Attributes of Medical Professional Judgement and Competence.* University of Sussex, Sussex. Reproduced at www.informatics.sussex.ac.uk/users/bend/doh

4 Fraser SW and Greenhalgh T (2001) Coping with complexity: educating for capability. *British Medical Journal.* **323:** 799–802.

5 General Medical Practice (2001) *Good Medical Practice.* General Medical Council, London.

6 Pendleton D, Schofield T, Tate P and Havelock P (2003) *The New Consultation, Developing Doctor–Patient Communication.* Oxford University Press, Oxford.

7 King J (2002) Career focus: 360° appraisal. *British Medical Journal.* **324:** S195.

8   Royal College of General Practitioners/General Practitioners Committee (2002) *Good Medical Practice for General Practitioners*. Royal College of General Practitioners, London.

9   National Institute for Clinical Excellence (NICE) www.nice.org.uk

10 Scottish Intercollegiate Guidelines Network (SIGN) www.sign.ac.uk

11 Irvine D and Irvine S (eds) (1991) *Making Sense of Audit*. Radcliffe Medical Press, Oxford.

12 Toon P, Greenhalgh T, Rigby M *et al.* (2002) *The Human Face of Medicine*. Two CD-ROMs in the APOLLO (Advancing Professional Practice through Online Learning Opportunities) series. BMJ Publishing Group, London. Free sample available at www.apollobmj.com

13 *Guidelines in Practice* www.eguidelines.co.uk

14 www.doctors.net.uk

15 www.npcrdc.man.ac.uk

16 www.ex.ac.uk/cfep

17 Department of Health (2003) *EPP Update newsletter*. Department of Health, London. See Expert Patient Programme on www.ohn.gov.uk/ohn/people/expert.htm

18 Department of Health (2004) *The NHS Knowledge and Skills Framework (NHS KSF) and Development Review Guidance – working draft*. Version 7. Department of Health, London.

19 Department of Health (2003) *Job Evaluation Handbook*. Version 1. Department of Health, London.

20 Chambers R, Drinkwater C and Boath E (2003) *Involving Patients and the Public: how to do it better* (2e). Radcliffe Medical Press, Oxford.

21 Mohanna K and Chambers R (2000) *Risk Matters in Healthcare*. Radcliffe Medical Press, Oxford.

22 Hart E and Fletcher J (1999) Learning how to change: a selective analysis of literature and experience of how teams learn and organisations change. *Journal of Interprofessional Care*. **13(1):** 53–63.

23 Maxwell RJ (1984) Quality assessment in health. *British Medical Journal*. **288:** 1470–2.

24 Firth-Cozens J (1993) *Audit in Mental Health Services*. LEA, Hove.

25 McCulloch D (2003) *Valuing Health in Practice*. Ashgate Publishing Ltd, Aldershot.

3

Demonstrating common components of good quality healthcare

In looking at the quality of care you provide and demonstrating your standards of service delivery and outcomes of learning, you should find that obtaining informed consent from patients for their treatment, maintaining confidentiality and handling complaints are part of the fabric of good quality care. We have considered them separately in this chapter, but each may be individualised to any of the seven clinical areas of Chapters 5 to 11.

We have set out the chapter with key information about consent followed by some example cycles of the stages of evidence (*see* Figure 1.1 on page 6). The two other sections on confidentiality and complaints follow, laid out in similar ways. Read through the cycles of evidence to become familiar with the approach to gathering and documenting evidence of your learning, competence, performance or standards of service delivery. Then either adopt one of the examples or adapt it to your own circumstances. Alternatively, read on to one or more of the clinical chapters and look at these three components in a clinical context such as in relation to arthritis (Chapter 7) or palliative care (Chapter 10).

Consent

Key points

Information given to a health professional remains the property of the patient. In most circumstances, consent is assumed for the necessary sharing of information with other professionals involved with the care of the patient for that episode of care. Usually consent is also assumed for essential sharing of information for continuing care. Beyond this, informed consent must be obtained. Patients attend for healthcare in the belief that the personal information that they supply, or which is found out about them during investigation or treatment, will be confidential.

Exceptions to the above are:[1]

- if the patient consents
- if it is in the patient's own interest that information should be disclosed, but it is either impossible to seek the patient's consent or
- it is medically undesirable in the patient's own interest, to seek the patient's consent
- if the law requires (and does not merely permit) the health professional to disclose the information
- if the health professional has an overriding duty to society to disclose the information
- if the health professional agrees with a governmental agency, that disclosure is necessary to safeguard national security
- if the disclosure is necessary to prevent a serious risk to public health
- in certain circumstances, for the purposes of medical research.

> Health professionals must be able to justify their decision to disclose information without consent. If they are in any doubt, they should consult their professional bodies and colleagues.

Consent is only valid if the patient fully understands the nature and consequences of disclosure – they must be able to give their consent, receive enough information to enable them to make a decision and be acting under their own free will and not persuaded by the strong influence of another person. If consent is given, the health worker is responsible for limiting the disclosure to that information for which informed consent has been obtained. The development of modern information technology and the increasing amount of multidisciplinary teamwork in patient care make confidentiality difficult to uphold.

You may need to give information about a patient to a relative or carer. Normally the consent of the patient should be obtained. Sometimes, the clinical condition of the patient may prevent informed consent being obtained (e.g. they are unconscious or have a severe illness). It is important to recognise that relatives or carers do not have any right to information about the patient. Disclosure without consent may be justified when third parties are exposed to a risk so serious that it outweighs the patient's privacy. An example would be if a patient declines to allow you to disclose information about their health and continues to drive against medical advice when unfit to do so.

Local research ethics committees and the research governance framework ensure best practice in the giving of informed consent by patients in research studies.

As health professionals, we often assume implied consent. The general public and patients are generally ignorant of the extent to which information about them is passed around the NHS. When teaching at both undergraduate and postgraduate levels, in examinations and assessments and in research, we may incorrectly assume patients imply their consent. Consent is also implied for health service accounting, central monitoring of referrals, in disease registers, for audit and in facilitating joint working between team members. The NHS is still engaged in a debate about what data can legitimately be shared without patients' explicit consent. Although written consent is usually obtained for supplying information to insurance companies or for legal reports, patients are often unaware of the type of information being supplied and have not given 'informed consent'. Guidelines published jointly by the British Medical Association (BMA) and the Association of British Insurers clarify that doctors are not required to release all aspects of a patient's medical history but need only submit (with the patient's consent) information that is relevant.[2]

The GMC's booklet *Seeking Patients' Consent: the ethical considerations* explores issues of consent in more depth and advises that:

> the amount of information you give each patient will vary according to factors such as the nature of the condition, the complexity of the treatment, the risks associated with the treatment or procedure and the patient's own wishes … you should be careful about relying on a patient's apparent compliance with a procedure as a form of consent.[3]

Collecting data to demonstrate your learning, competence, performance and standards of service delivery: consent

Example cycle of evidence 3.1

- Focus: informed consent
- Other relevant focus: research

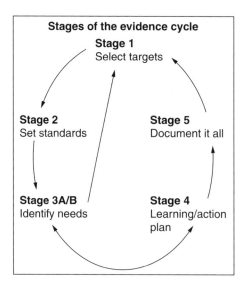

Stages of the evidence cycle

Stage 1
Select targets

Stage 2
Set standards

Stage 5
Document it all

Stage 3A/B
Identify needs

Stage 4
Learning/action plan

Case study 3.1

You agree as a practice to undertake a survey to find out if patients are satisfied with your service. The practice manager will organise it, but you are nominated to lead the work. You decide to focus on teenagers as a group as the adolescent drop-in clinic you set up two years ago with the school health service is not being used as much as it once was. You want to be proactive about helping teenagers resist smoking and drugs, encourage healthy eating and exercise, protect their mental health and encourage their management of chronic diseases such as asthma and diabetes, etc. You are not sure how to survey the teenagers. You think they are unlikely to answer questionnaires sent through the post and think you will interview teenagers about their satisfaction with the clinic. You intend to employ one of your own teenage children to interview some who have never come to the clinic, by selecting their names from your patient list as well as some teenagers who have attended. You're not sure if you are getting into research territory or if it is okay to claim you are auditing your services.

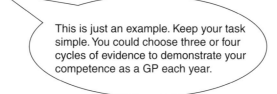

This is just an example. Keep your task simple. You could choose three or four cycles of evidence to demonstrate your competence as a GP each year.

Stage 1: Select your aspirations for good practice

The excellent GP:

- protects patients' rights and makes sure that they are not disadvantaged by taking part in research
- gives patients the information they need about their problem in a way they can understand as a basis for informed consent.

Stage 2: Set the standards for your outcomes

Outcomes might include:

- the way learning is applied
- a learnt skill
- a protocol
- a strategy that is implemented
- meeting recommended standards.

- The informed consent policy of the practice covers patients' participation in audit and research as well as consent to clinical treatment.
- You are able to describe the difference between what is audit of clinical management and service provision and what is research.

Stage 3A: Identify your learning needs

- Read through the frequently asked questions and answers on the Department of Health website relating to research governance.[4] Consider whether you are able to answer the questions before reading the answers.

- Describe an audit plan of an adolescent clinic that involves obtaining young people's views of standards of services by interviewing them. Submit the plan to the chair of the local research ethics committee to check that he/she agrees that the audit proposal does not fall within the definition of research and to approve the patient literature and the process inviting informed consent to take part.
- Self-assess your own knowledge about teenagers consenting to treatment or research, and identify any differences in your approach if they are under or over the age of 16 years.

Stage 3B: Identify your service needs

Any of the needs assessment exercises in 3A may also reveal service needs.

- Draw up an information leaflet for young people about the audit of adolescent clinic services that you intend to carry out. Ask others to critique the leaflet – young people for its readability and clarity, a research colleague for the extent to which it conforms to best practice for informed consent. Use the information leaflet so that they can give informed consent to the interview to obtain their views and an audio recording of the interview.
- Ask a colleague to peer review the extent to which advice and information you give to teenagers during a consultation is accurate. The teenager would need to have given prior, written informed consent for the peer review (and audio recording if used).

Stage 4: Make and carry out a learning and action plan

- Obtain and read the documents about research governance from the Department of Health's website or from your PCO – as in the first point in section 3A.[4]
- Study the application form for the ethical approval of a research study.
- Understand the limits to obtaining patients' views as part of audit of clinical and service management by reading up on informed consent. Read the GMC's booklet: *Seeking Patients' Consent: the ethical considerations.*[3] Look at whether you are explaining the details of the diagnosis or prognosis, giving an explanation of likely benefits and side-effects, explaining whether a proposed treatment is experimental and whether a doctor in training will be involved.
- Ask for a short tutorial from your local clinical governance lead about good practice in obtaining patients' views through audit, research and patient involvement activities – including good practice in informed consent and any special considerations for teenagers aged under 16 years.

Stage 5: Document your learning, competence, performance and standards of service delivery

- Keep a comparison of your own practice with the answers to the frequently asked questions on the Department of Health website relating to research governance.[4]
- File a copy of the response letter from the chair of local research ethics committee about the audit proposal.
- Document that the subsequent revised audit plan shows that the work does not fall within the definition of research.
- Keep a copy of the revised teenage patients' informed consent leaflet, following the critique.
- Repeat the peer review by the same, or another colleague, of the extent to which advice and information you give to teenagers during consultations is accurate.

Case study 3.1 continued

The chair of the research ethics committee advises you that your plan should be classed as research rather than audit as it involves contact with patients outside their usual NHS care. He explains about the risks of using untrained interviewers such as your own children, and the need to fully inform those teenagers you are inviting to be interviewed about the survey and that their refusal will not prejudice their medical care. He advises you to send an application form for formal approval to the ethics committee and to contact the research lead in your PCO in line with the research governance framework if you wish to continue to develop a research project. You revise your plans as the scale of the work required is becoming out of all proportion.

Confidentiality

Key points

You should have appropriate confidentiality safeguards in place in the practice to prevent inadvertent disclosure of personal and sensitive information about patients. Tell people, especially the young, about their right to confidential medical treatment and reinforce your conversation with posters and leaflets. People with non-prescription drug-related problems who seek help from substance abuse clinics, or those with sexually transmitted infections who attend genitourinary medicine clinics, often do not want their GP to be told because they do not believe that the information will be kept confidential. Fears about confidentiality are the commonest reason young people give for not attending their GP for contraceptive treatment.[5]

Young people under the age of 16 years have the same rights to confidentiality as other patients. The younger the person, the greater care is needed to assess the level of understanding to ensure that he or she understands the consequences of any proposed action. If a young person fulfils the conditions of the Fraser Guidelines (England and Wales) he or she is regarded as being competent to make his or her own decisions.[6] In Scotland, the Age of Legal Capacity (Scotland) Act 1991 gives similar powers of consent to those under 16 years of age. In Northern Ireland separate legislation applies. The Fraser Guidelines are included within the *Best Practice Guidance for Doctors and Other Health Professionals on the Provision of Advice and Treatment to Young People under 16 on Contraception, Sexual and Reproductive Health* published by the Department of Health in July 2004.[6]

Occasionally you may feel that you have a moral obligation to divulge confidential information. Whenever possible you should seek to persuade the patient to give consent to the disclosure. Seek advice from your professional organisations in circumstances where others are at danger (e.g. risk of harm, or rape or sexual abuse), or where a serious crime has been committed. Health professionals should satisfy themselves that sufficient authority has been obtained (e.g. a certificate from the Attorney General or Lord Advocate) and consult professional organisations before disclosing information without a patient's consent.

The Caldicott Committee Report described principles of good practice to safeguard confidentiality when information is being used for non-clinical purposes:[7]

- justify the purpose
- do not use patient-identifiable information unless it is absolutely necessary
- use the minimum necessary patient-identifiable information
- access to patient-identifiable information should be on a strict need-to-know basis
- everyone with access to patient-identifiable information should be aware of his or her responsibilities.

Interpreters should be used wherever possible to avoid the use of friends or relatives. They should be trained in the requirements of confidentiality.

Patients are entitled to access data held about them. Exceptions to this right are:

- the patient failed to make the request in accordance with the Data Protection Act 1998
- if acceding to the request would result in disclosure of information about somebody else without their consent

- when giving medical information may cause serious harm to the mental or physical health of the patient (a rare occurrence).

You need to incorporate systems for ensuring that paper and computer security are maintained. Systems for monitoring and upgrading security systems should be in place and you should check regularly that confidentiality is not being breached if changes are made.

Collecting data to demonstrate your learning, competence, performance and standards of service delivery: confidentiality

Example cycle of evidence 3.2

- Focus: confidentiality
- Other relevant focus: teaching and training

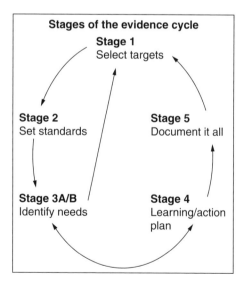

Stages of the evidence cycle

Stage 1
Select targets

Stage 2
Set standards

Stage 5
Document it all

Stage 3A/B
Identify needs

Stage 4
Learning/action plan

Case study 3.2

It is the first time you have had medical students placed with you and you want to teach two of them about the importance of making sure that student visitors understand the practice code on confidentiality while they are on their placement with you.

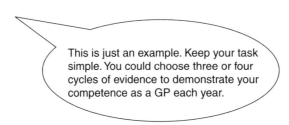

This is just an example. Keep your task simple. You could choose three or four cycles of evidence to demonstrate your competence as a GP each year.

Stage 1: Select your aspirations for good practice

The excellent GP:

- maintains the confidentiality of patient-specific information
- ensures that patients are not put at risk when seeing students or doctors in training.

Stage 2: Set the standards for your outcomes

Outcomes might include:

- the way learning is applied
- a learnt skill
- a protocol
- a strategy that is implemented
- meeting recommended standards.

- Ensure that all members of the practice team including you, new members of staff and students or doctors in training, are familiar with guidelines for confidentiality in relation to patients receiving healthcare.

Stage 3A: Identify your learning needs

- Assess your knowledge about the limits of confidentiality, e.g. for providing help for under-16 year olds with a drug problem or divulging information about the health of patients with cancer to relatives or carers.
- Ask an expert tutor's opinion about the particular method of teaching you plan to use for an in-house training session. The session will be on maintaining confidentiality for teenagers of different ages and people with life-threatening health problems. It should convey the main messages and lead to changes where necessary.

Stage 3B: Identify your service needs

Any of the needs assessment exercises in 3A may also reveal service needs.

- Compare the practice protocol for confidentiality with the guidelines in the *Confidentiality and Young People* toolkit.[5]
- Review your current or the intended induction programme for new members of staff, students on placement and doctors in training, to assess the extent to which knowledge of confidentiality features and is addressed.
- Organise a test of several different examples of patient episodes for members of the practice team, where confidentiality is complex and students or staff may be uncertain about the correct approach, based on the frequently asked questions on confidentiality published by the GMC.[8,9]

Stage 4: Make and carry out a learning and action plan

- Find out from the local educational tutor how to undertake learning needs assessments of others from different disciplines with different levels of responsibilities in respect of confidentiality.
- Prepare for and run an interactive teaching session on confidentiality for patients of all age groups and conditions. You might invite the whole practice team, including students, family planning or school nurses, local pharmacists, GP registrars, etc. You could use the *Confidentiality and Young People* toolkit and the answers to the GMC's frequently asked questions, for promoting discussion with the practice team at the session.[5,8,9]

Stage 5: Document your learning, competence, performance and standards of service delivery

- Keep the answers of the quiz completed by those attending the teaching session before and after their training about confidentiality.
- Keep an incident record kept by the practice team of any reported or perceived breaches of confidentiality by anyone working in, or associated with, the practice.
- Include examples of personal learning plans based on learning needs assessments for new staff or doctors in training by the end of their induction period.
- Include the revised practice protocol in line with the *Confidentiality and Young People* toolkit and GMC guidance on confidentiality.[5,8,9]

Case study 3.2 continued

Other staff colleagues join your teaching session with the students using the video from the *Confidentiality and Young People* toolkit.[5] All get full marks in the quiz after watching the video. The frequently asked questions published by the GMC really enhance their understanding about how confidentiality issues are managed in practice.[8,9]

Learning from complaints

Key points

There is learning to be had from every complaint. The GMC received a record 5539 complaints in 2002, 4% more than in 2001; of these, 72 resulted in a doctor being banned or suspended.[10] Even if the complaint is trivial or undeserved, it implies a lack of communication. Table 3.1 describes the nature of claims against GPs reported in a study of 1000 consecutive clinical cases. There are a myriad of associated reasons for the claims. Many of the clinical events will reveal failings in the practice systems and processes and in the practice of the GP – such as communication, diagnostic skills, etc.

Table 3.1: Nature of 1000 claims against GPs handled by the Medical Protection Society[11]

Claim by patient	Number of claims
Problems of diagnosis (delayed or missed)	631
Prescribing errors	193
Malignant neoplasms (some of the problems of diagnosis)	140
Cancer of the breast (lumpiness often falsely diagnosed as benign)	20
Cancer of the cervix (often abnormalities are filed away and not acted upon)	14
Cancer of the digestive organs (cancer of colon most frequent with misdiagnosed symptoms)	21
Diabetes (8 deaths) primary failure to diagnose (19 delays in diagnosis; 9 delays in referral of patient resulting in amputation)	40
Myocardial infarction 27 deaths (8 undiagnosed, 7 diagnosed as dyspepsia; 3 diagnosed as congestive cardiac failure; 3 as muscular origin; 2 as chest infection)	34
Prescribing	
Steroids (e.g. osteoporotic collapse)	40
Antibiotic allergy	8
Phenothiazines (extrapyramidal symptoms)	10
Hormone replacement therapy	9
Oral contraception	9
Warfarin (interactions e.g. resulting in cerebral haemorrhage)	5

Collecting data to demonstrate your learning, competence, performance and standards of service delivery: complaints

Example cycle of evidence 3.3

- Focus: complaints
- Other relevant focus: working with colleagues

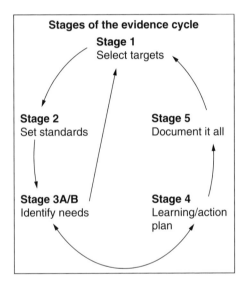

Stages of the evidence cycle

Stage 1
Select targets

Stage 2
Set standards

Stage 5
Document it all

Stage 3A/B
Identify needs

Stage 4
Learning/action plan

Case study 3.3

Your practice has received a patient complaint about a GP locum failing to suspect a patient's secondary cancer on the first occasion they consulted with back pain. This has prompted you all as a practice team to review the way that your complaints system functions.

This is just an example. Keep your task simple. You could choose three or four cycles of evidence to demonstrate your competence as a GP each year.

Stage 1: Select your aspirations for good practice

The excellent GP:

- apologises appropriately when things go wrong, and has an adequate complaints procedure in place.

Stage 2: Set the standards for your outcomes

Outcomes might include:

- the way learning is applied
- a learnt skill
- a protocol
- a strategy that is implemented
- meeting recommended standards.

- Understand and establish effective processes for preventing and managing complaints from patients in the practice.

Stage 3A: Identify your learning needs

- Examine as a significant event one or more complaints, e.g. where the practice has not advised a patient correctly about the complaints process.
- Compare the actual care of a patient against an acceptable standard of care for a range of clinical conditions as ongoing review for clinical area that has been the subject of a complaint (e.g. back pain in the case study). You could use peer review by asking respected colleagues, or compare your practice against a published standard such as a guideline by a responsible body of professional opinion.

Stage 3B: Identify your service needs

Any of the needs assessment exercises in 3A may also reveal service needs.

- Audit patient complaints in the preceding 12 months: the number, the outcomes and how the complaint system is advertised, etc.
- Audit the extent to which doctors and nurses are following practice agreed protocols. Be proactive about preventing or minimising the likelihood of the source of the complaint recurring.

- Audit vulnerable areas. Look back at the analysis of complaints to identify useful areas for focusing learning, e.g. a review of the prescribing of steroids.
- Review the way that the qualifications of locums are checked and that they are made aware of the practice protocols.

Stage 4: Make and carry out a learning and action plan

- Ask your PCO to look at the practice complaints system and feed back how it can be improved (if at all).
- Arrange a tutorial between the practice manager and others in the team about preventing and managing complaints, or use one of the risk management packages produced by medical defence organisations.[12,13]
- Read up on how to undertake significant event analysis including how to share the information with the practice team and respond as a practice team.

Stage 5: Document your learning, competence, performance and standards of service delivery

- Include evidence of clinical competence to guard against a complaint.
- Include the protocol of the patient complaint process against which consecutive complaints can be audited in another 12 months' time.
- Record the guidance about physical examinations, including that the reason for any examination should be communicated clearly, that a chaperone should be offered for any internal or breast examination, and the comfort and privacy of the patient should always be kept in mind to avoid potential complaints.
- Record that a file containing practice protocols is available for easy reference on the desktop of the computer.

Case study 3.3 continued

You are invited by your PCO to take a lead in advising GPs in other practices about the handling of complaints because they were impressed by the way your complaint system was applied when you invited them to visit your practice and advise about the handling of complaints.

References

1 Chambers R and Wakley G (2000) *Making Clinical Governance Work for You.* Radcliffe Medical Press, Oxford.

2 British Medical Association and Association of British Insurers (2002) *Medical Information and Insurance.* British Medical Association, London. See www. bma.org.uk/ap.nsf/Content/MedicalInfoInsurance

3 General Medical Council (2002) *Seeking Patients' Consent: the ethical consider-ations.* General Medical Council, London.

4 www.dh.gov.uk/PolicyAnd Guidance/ResearchAnd Development/fs/en

5 Royal College of General Practitioners and Brook (2000) *Confidentiality and Young People. A toolkit for general practice, primary care groups and trusts.* Royal College of General Practitioners, London.

6 http://www.dh.gov.uk/assetRoot/04/08/69/14/04086914.pdf

7 Department of Health (1997) Report of the review of patient-identifiable infor-mation. In: *The Caldicott Committee Report.* Department of Health, London.

8 General Medical Council (2004) *Confidentiality: protecting and providing infor-mation.* General Medical Council, London.

9 General Medical Council (2004) *Frequently Asked Questions. Confidentiality: protecting and providing information.* General Medical Council, London. See www.gmc-uk.org for updated questions and answers.

10 General Medical Council (2003) *Fitness to Practise Statistics for 2002.* General Medical Council, London.

11 Panting G (2003) *Nature of 1000 Claims against GPs.* Medical Protection Society, London (presentation at primary care conference, Birmingham).

12 MPS Risk Consulting, Granary Wharf House, Leeds LS11 5PY or www.mps-riskconsulting.com

13 MDU Services Ltd, 230 Blackfriars Road, London SE1 8PJ or www.the-mdu.com

4

Providing high-quality care as a general practitioner with special clinical interest in drug misuse

Deciding to provide a service for drug abusers

The national enhanced service funds practices to:

- develop and co-ordinate the care of drug users, and develop practice guidelines
- treat dependent drug users with support
- ensure that prescribing takes place within a context in which the co-existing physical, emotional, social and legal problems are addressed as far as possible
- participate in audits of prescribing practice
- act as a resource to practice colleagues in the care of drug misusers
- demonstrate additional training and continuing professional development
- maintain the safety and training of clinical and non-clinical staff
- provide care for patients outside their own registered list if the practice has agreed to do so.

The role as a GP with a special interest

The NHS Plans for England, Scotland, Wales and Northern Ireland identified the need to create a new role for GPs, called a practitioner with special clinical interest (GPwSI).[1] The Department of Health commissioned the RCGP to identify the skills, knowledge and experience required for practitioners to be competent to work in this position.[2] The RCGP drew heavily on work produced by the RCGP National Experts' Group in Drug Training, a group that has been instrumental in developing the training for GPwSIs in drug misuse. A GPwSI will be expected to act as an interim level of expertise, support and advice for local colleagues and the PCO.

What is a GPwSI?

Most GPs have a special interest in one area or another. Many of you may be involved in education, perhaps are trainers; some of you may have a lead role within your PCO and others may do sessions in local family planning services or within other community (or indeed acute trust) settings. Perhaps what distinguishes a GPwSI from these roles, though, is that a GPwSI would be expected to provide an 'enhanced' service, usually outside the confines of their practice and act independently. The RCGP and the Department of Health define a GPwSI as a doctor who is qualified and competent, through undertaking specific training, to provide not only the full range of generalist service but also those defined by the special interest service. Different models will be developed according to local need, though in all circumstances clinical accountability rests with the GPwSI who is responsible for his or her actions, including referral to specialist care and the need to work with other professional groups where appropriate. Overall accountability rests with the employing or contracting authority.

Quintessential to being a GP is that the doctor works independently of direct supervision. This may include accepting referrals, making diagnosis, supervising or administering treatment, and discharging from care or running a care programme for specific conditions. A GPwSI could be said to extend this means of working beyond the confines of their practice.

Working as a GPwSI does not mean working in isolation from related acute trust services, with whom GPwSIs may associate in a common venue, share clinical governance activities, and participate in joint organisation and professional development when appropriate (*see* Box 4.1).

Box 4.1:   Definition of a GP with special clinical interest[1]

A GPwSI is a GP with appropriate experience, able to independently deliver a service, working in a clinical area outside the normal remit of general practice care, with a fair contract in respect of terms and conditions of service and annual leave entitlement, in an appropriate venue, working within a defined quality framework and able to accept referrals from GPs and other professional colleagues.

As a GPwSI, you should be seen as one option available to your PCO for service delivery, and must be part of a co-ordinated approach to treatment services and not merely be seen as a pragmatic solution to dealing with waiting lists. It is important that as a GPwSI you are not viewed as a substitute to a specialist service. Where a specialist provider is not in place then your PCO must ensure that a suitably trained practitioner fills this gap, rather than using the GPwSI as a substitute. This is vital if the level of specialist opinion is to be maintained rather than risking diluting the number and expertise of practitioners able to provide this specialist input.

What should a GPwSI in drug misuse do?

Your activities in providing the GPwSI service will vary according to local need, your skills and competencies and other local factors. Service providers and user organisations as well as representatives from the PCO should ideally be involved in the planning stages of the service.

The following are examples of core activities of a GPwSI service.

Clinical service

Provide a clinical service for patients with drug misuse (*see* Box 4.2). These services can be offered as

- part of an integrated general practice service with care being provided alongside other general medical services (GMS, PMS or PMS plus)
- a stand-alone service located within a dedicated drug misuse service within the NHS (primary or secondary care) or other provider:
  - targeted to a particular population or risk group (e.g. pregnant users, hard-to-reach groups)
  - provided as part of a generic drug misuse service.

Box 4.2:   Opportunities to provide clinical care

- Within the GP surgery: providing extra or advanced services to special population of patients or to larger numbers.
- Within a specialist drug misuse service: providing primary care expertise alongside drug treatment.
- Within a homeless hostel, prison or other secure environment.

Education and liaison

- In partnership with others, support the development of training for GPs and GP registrars in drug misuse.

- Provide information and support to practices and practitioners on best practice in relation to care of illegal drug-using patients.
- Provide a bridge between primary and specialist addiction services.

Leadership

- Develop pathways of care for patients with drug problems, including the development of local referral and treatment guidance.
- Develop clinical capacity for patients in primary care, as part of either local or nationally enhanced services, as defined in the GMS contract.
- Support the development of harm reduction across the PCO.

What skills and experience should I have?

The minimum standards are those outlined within the Drug Misuse Clinical Guidelines.[3] All GPwSIs should meet these minimum standards before providing a GPwSI service. The RCGP has developed a 'foundation'-based course to meet the requirements of the generalist practitioner. This includes the core competencies for nurses, pharmacists and the GP performing as a 'generalist' in the care, treatment and management of a drug-using patient in primary care that will underpin the foundation to the certificate course. The core competencies have been selected from the Drug and Alcohol National Occupational Standards and the standards required of a GP providing a national enhanced service under the GMS contract. As a GPwSI, you would be expected to provide safe, evidence-based care to drug users, beyond the generalist level – to an intermediate level of expertise.

A GPwSI in drug misuse would be expected to be competent at providing the following.

Clinical service

Have a good understanding of the treatment of drug users as laid out in the National Drug Misuse Clinical Guidelines,[3] in particular:

- be able to provide safe, evidence-based interventions to drug users, including those with less co-morbidity[a] across a range of commonly used substances, and using a range of commonly used treatment interventions including pharmacological interventions (e.g. methadone mixture, buprenorphine, lofexidine, naltrexone), psychological interventions (brief interventions, problem-solving motivational interviewing), and an understanding of the range of social interventions available

[a]Severe co-morbidity would include patients with serious personality disorders and other serious mental health problems, physical problems such as liver failure, and serious social problems.

- a sound understanding of harm reduction interventions in relation to drug misuse.

Education and liaison

- A sound understanding of the legal framework underpinning drug misuse.
- A good knowledge of local educational opportunities and funding in relation to drug misuse training.
- A good understanding of different professional roles in relation to drug users.
- An ability to work in a multidisciplinary team.
- Knowledge of local drug action team priorities or other commissioning organisations or structures.

Leadership

- Good negotiating skills.
- Good communication skills.
- A sound understanding of the local and national policies that underpin the treatment of drug users in the UK.
- Sound understanding of current local and national primary care policy in relation to the treatment of drug users.

As a GPwSI it is important that you are able to recognise the limitations of your knowledge and competencies in the drug misuse area and are aware of when and how to refer patients to other services. You would be expected to work in collaboration with community-based nurses and, where relevant, community pharmacists in shared care of drug users across a geographical area. You would be expected to participate in your local commissioning process and have a broad understanding of the concept of needs assessment, service development planning, and the roles and responsibilities of others involved in service planning. You would be expected to be competent at providing primary care leadership to your PCO in drug misuse.

How can I obtain these skills and experience?

As a generalist

PCOs will need to ensure that you are first and foremost a competent and experienced generalist, as well as having the specific competencies and experience for the special interest area. This can be assessed in a number of ways but is readily demonstrated by GPs who have passed the Membership Examination of the Royal College of General Practitioners (MRCGP) and who are current members of the College. There are other ways; these will involve you collecting evidence to show that you are a competent generalist – look at the headings of the RCGP's *Good Medical Practice for General Practitioners*.[4,5]

By having a special interest

Beyond this it is recommended that you show:

- evidence of relevant experience such as that you are able to demonstrate competencies against core activities
- demonstrable experience working with drug users such that you are able to provide care that adheres to the standards outlined in the Department of Health Drug Misuse Clinical Guidelines.[3] Ideally, at least some of this experience needs to be in a community setting and under direct supervision from a specialist (the specialist may be a consultant addiction specialist or experienced GP working with drug users). It is expected that you are able to demonstrate experience managing patients across a variety of differing substances (e.g. heroin addicts, cannabis and stimulant users), and that you have experience using a number of different treatment interventions. This chapter outlines some examples in Table 4.1
- evidence of attendance at relevant courses or self directed learning to meet learning gaps identified through the professional development plan. The RCGP holds an annual conference aimed at bringing together primary care practitioners from a range of disciplines to examine current practice and recent advances in the field (*see* Box 4.3). This conference offers opportunities to develop a learning network that will offer support as you work as a GPwSI.

Box 4.3:   Certificate in Drug Misuse

The RCGP has established a Certificate in Drug Misuse, which is a 6-day mentor-led training programme involving course work and assessments.[6,7] The course has undergone an accreditation process and is quality assured through an overarching National Experts' Advisory Group made up of senior representation from relevant stakeholders. In addition, the RCGP runs a number of kite-marked Special Interest Master Classes to address other learning needs.

Table 4.1: Examples of evidence to meet criteria as a GPwSI

Good medical practice: able to provide safe evidence-based interventions for a whole range of substance misuse problems e.g.

- Documentation of at least one clinical audit of management of substance misuse in your service.
- Details of services provided by you or supervised by you.
- Details of local clinical or good practice guidelines/guidance or protocols.
- Details of your clinical care development needs.
- Details of care pathways and referral routes for patients that you are asked to see on behalf of your colleagues or that you are unable to manage yourself and need to refer to specialist colleagues.
- Details of the factors in your workplace or more widely that may constrain you in the delivery of high-quality evidence-based care – this may include policies within your organisation such as non-use of methadone as the drug of choice in the treatment of drug users, constraints on dosages used, etc.

Maintaining good medical practice: able to demonstrate a sound understanding of the educational opportunities and funding in relation to substance misuse training, e.g.

- Give details of courses/conferences/master classes, and evidence that you have attended these for at least nine hours per year.
- Evidence of updating skills in relation to new pharmacological treatments.
- Evidence of maintaining skills in psychological interventions.
- Evidence of maintaining skills in relevant practice procedures (this may be relevant to doctors working predominately in a clinical setting providing direct clinical care alongside drug misuse treatment, such as a homeless hostel).

Relationship with patients: able to demonstrate how you ensure communication and involvement with patients, e.g.

- Evidence of significant event analysis in relation to your drug treatment service, including all drug-related deaths (or near misses) within your service.
- Examples of leaflets and information you provide for your drug misuse service.

Working with colleagues: able to demonstrate how you build and maintain good working relationships with your colleagues, e.g.

- Description of the team and/or managerial structures in which you work.
- Evidence that demonstrates a good understanding of the roles of professional groups in relation to drug users; this may involve undertaking a joint consultation with another professional, examining care pathways together, etc.
- Evidence of working with other professionals and agencies.
- Evidence of undertaking or participating in a community care assessment.

Teaching and training, e.g.

- Present a summary of formal teaching and training delivered external to your organisation.
- Details of formal mentor or education supervision.
- Details of undertaking an extended case study.

continued

Probity: what safeguards are in place to ensure propriety in the managerial and financial aspects of your specialist role?

- Evidence of correct handling of payments for research and/or educational activities.
- Examples of where the doctor–patient relationship may be blurred.

Management activities

- Describe your role on the drug action team or other PCO umbrella organisation with respect to commissioning drug services.
- Describe positions you hold on local or national committees.

Research

- Show evidence of research proposals or outlines of areas of study.
- Evidence of articles published or being prepared.

Health

- Mention any problems you may have with respect to your own health issues.

How can I demonstrate that I have the necessary competencies to work as a GPwSI?

Since 2003, you will have had to undergo an annual appraisal and should be well versed in the use of a PDP to both record your professional development and help to identify your learning needs. Your PDP should also be used as your special interest portfolio – preferably together with your generalist work. This portfolio should form part of your GPwSI annual appraisal and contain examples of evidence to show that you have obtained and maintained the competencies described in this chapter (*see* section on appraisal, page 3).

What about appraisal?

Each practitioner is required to undergo an annual appraisal, the mechanism approved by each individual PCO. In addition, there is a recommendation that the appraiser has in-depth or specialist knowledge of the GP's special interest area, this person usually being the local specialist consultant. This may be a suitable mechanism where there is a close relationship between the GPwSI and the specialist service, for example, where the GPwSI works alongside an acute sector service. However, it will not suit many other areas where an equivalent secondary care service may not exist, such as the care of the homeless, prison medicine, or where the GPwSI provides a service far removed from the acute or mental health trust equivalent such as primary care drug misuse. For these clinicians, ways need to be introduced for accreditation, appraisal and re-validation that ensure that the doctor is fit to practise.

The appraisal process

The appraisal process must embrace the generalist and special interest elements of your work.[8] Where relevant, your special interest and generalist skills would be appraised during the same appraisal process. The RCGP National Experts' Advisory Group recommends that all GPwSIs in drug misuse undertake an appraisal focusing on their special interest area at least once in a five-year revalidation cycle, and that a practitioner with an in-depth knowledge of the special interest area undertakes this appraisal. In this case, there is an expectation that the appraiser would have an in-depth knowledge of the special interest area. In some areas, there may be no local specialist available to take on the appraisal, or where the special interest area crosses current boundaries of primary care/specialist services, there may not be an equivalent 'expert' at all. In these cases, the PCO will be required to identify an appraiser/supervisor from another area, or from a national resource. These can be drawn from a national pool, as with the RCGP National Drug Misuse Training Team regional clinical leads or from identifying a peer working in a similar role.

What about continuing professional development?

The RCGP's National Experts' Advisory Group on drug misuse training has recommended that in the year following appointment as a GPwSI in drug abuse you undertake a programme of CPD in drug misuse. The exact contact should be defined and determined by your learning needs though ideally should be at least nine hours per year.

What if I want to continue my training and become a specialist?

As yet there is no agreed or defined means to becoming a specialist practitioner via general practice, though there is every reason that GPs can develop the necessary skills, experience and knowledge and can in the future be employed to lead clinical services. In the field of drug misuse many GPs already lead services, undertake research and development and are paid by their PCO for providing what amounts to a GP consultant service. Though this has developed, it has in general been in an ad-hoc means with confusion as to where the boundaries between the generalist-GPwSI-specialist are. The Drug Misuse Clinical Guidelines define a specialist as a practitioner who provides expertise, training and competence in drug misuse treatment as their main clinical activity. Such a practitioner works in a specialist multidisciplinary team, can carry out assessments of any case with complex needs and provide a full range of treatments and access to rehabilitation options. Most specialists would normally, but not always, be consultant psychiatrists who hold a Certificate of Completion of Specialist Training (CCST) in psychiatry and are therefore able to provide expertise, training and competence in drug misuse treatment as their main clinical activity. Their practice would probably involve the prescription of injectable and other specialised forms of prescribing and they can act as a resource in shared care arrangements for other practitioners and professional staff. They would be required to maintain their level of competence by attending appropriate training events.

The following is presented for discussion as a means for GPs not entering this area via the psychiatric route to become specialists.

Entry criteria

The doctor must have completed higher medical training in general medicine, general practice or public health medicine with an appropriate certificate of completion of higher medical training.

Core practical training and experience

- Details of elements of specialist areas of work as defined by the job plan including evidence of autonomous clinical practice and details of access to appropriate levels of clinical supervision.
- An attachment to a regional drug dependence unit, with outpatient and inpatient facilities.
- Two attachments to different community drug teams.
- An attachment to a community alcohol team and a regional alcohol unit with assessment and inpatient facilities.

Theoretical training

Attend or have registered to attend one of the following (minimum of two of these during the training period):

- a recognised diploma, masters or higher course in addiction studies or equivalent (e.g. study in patients in secure environments, homelessness)
- a nationally recognised leadership programme e.g. National Treatment Agency for substance misuse (NTA) leadership programme,[9] or NHS modernisation leadership course
- a recognised conference and/or course (minimum of one during the training programme), for example:
  - the annual Society for the Study of Addiction conference
  - the Royal College of Psychiatrists' Faculty of Substance Misuse annual conference
  - the annual Northern Specialist in Drug Dependence meeting
  - the annual RCGP primary care conference on the management of drug misusers
- quarterly meetings of the regional Clinicians with an Interest in Addiction (minimum four times during the training programme).

Process

Stage 1: baseline appraisal conducted by recognised appraiser. The main outcome of this activity will be the development of a learning plan and learning contract, detailing the learning and summative assessment process to enable the GP to meet the criteria and standards of a specialist provider.

Stage 2: assessment. The assessment will consist of the following:

- submission of the learning portfolio within the designated timescale
- satisfactory completion of the learning contract in order to achieve recognised specialist status (the method of evaluation is an appraisal and review of learning portfolio by the assessment panel)
- attendance at a viva involving a panel jointly approved by the RCGP National Experts' Advisory Group and the Royal College of Psychiatrists (RCP), perhaps involving the doctor, their supervising consultant nominated by the National Experts' Advisory Group and an external assessor.

Stage 3: approval. Recognition of specialist status by both the RCGP and the RCP.

Conclusion

As PCOs employ more GPwSIs to meet service needs, it is important that there is in place a robust system for these practitioners to develop and demonstrate their skills, knowledge and expertise. It is the responsibility of each individual doctor to be able to show that they are competent to undertake the roles and responsibility that they have been employed to provide within any given service. This is best done through the vehicle of a PDP and entering a cycle of lifelong learning.

References

1   www.dh.gov.uk

2   Department of Health Guidelines for the appointment of general practitioners with special interests in the delivery of clinical services in drug misuse. www.dh.gov.uk/assetRoot/04/08/28/64/04082864.pdf

3   Department of Health, The Scottish Office Department of Health, Welsh Office, Department of Health and Social Services, Northern Ireland (1999) Drug Misuse and Dependence – guidelines on clinical management. The Stationery Office, London. www.dh.gov.uk/assetRoot/04/07/81/98/04078198.pdf

4   General Medical Council (2001) *Good Medical Practice*. General Medical Council, London.

5   Royal College of General Practitioners/General Practitioners Committee (2002) *Good Medical Practice for General Practitioners*. Royal College of General Practitioners, London.

6   Gerada C and Murnane M (2003) *Drugs: Education, Prevention and Policy*. Royal College of General Practitioners' Certificate in Drug Misuse. **10**: 369–78.

7   Royal College of General Practitioners' Certificate in Drug Misuse, www.rcgp.org.uk/drug/certificate.asp

8   Department of Health The NHS Plan – a progress report www.dh.gov.uk/assetRoot/04/08/18/72/04081872.pdf

9   www.nta.nhs.uk

5

Illegal drug abuse

This chapter highlights some of the important areas about illegal drug abuse that GPs encounter in their everyday work. Chapter 4 gives advice on suitable training courses and how practices might provide enhanced or advanced services for people with drug abuse problems. Abuse of prescribed drugs is covered in Chapter 11.

Under the new contract for GPs, protection against hepatitis B, management of immediate referral, complications of drug abuse and acute withdrawal can be categorised as activities under core management. Advanced and enhanced services, provided by some practices with a special interest or need, are described in the previous chapter.

Evidence about illegal drugs can be found from various governmental publications.[1–3] The British Crime Survey in 1995 reported that 28% of 16–59 year olds had tried an illegal drug at least once.[3] The earliest age at which young people were likely to experiment with drugs was 12–13 years, with drug taking being most common among young adults in their late teens and early twenties. Around one-half of young people had tried a drug by their 20th birthday. Cannabis was the most widely taken illegal drug. The other significant trend was the growth in 'dance drugs'. These are largely confined to young adults under 25 years old, with lifetime use of ecstasy ranging from around 3% to 10%, with amphetamines and LSD consistently more popular than ecstasy. However, prevalence just means that people have tried drugs, and can give a misleading and alarmist impression of both the scale of everyday drug-taking behaviour and its effects. Some people will try a drug such as cannabis once, wonder what all the fuss was about and move on to more important things in life. At the other end of the scale, smaller numbers will develop drug-related problems and dependence, with their damaging effects on health, on personal or family relationships and on crime rates. Statistics from the report give an overview (*see* Box 5.1).[1]

Box 5.1:   Statistics relating to drug use[1]

- Lifetime experience of drugs is over 1 in 4 of the adult population in the UK. It is at its highest for 16–19 year-olds (46%) and 20–29 year olds (41%) and decreases in higher age groups to 12% for 50–59 year olds.
- Perhaps as many as 7 million people in the UK have tried cannabis at some point in their lives, while 250 000–800 000 young people may have tried ecstasy.
- Cannabis is more likely to be used frequently, with 9% of all cannabis users reporting daily use, and 14% taking it several times a week. Very few ecstasy, LSD and amphetamines users take these drugs daily, but about 20% take them more than monthly.
- Overall, at least 6% of the population (around 3 million people) will have used cannabis in the last 12 months. Among young people, around 1 in 5 use drugs on a regular (monthly) basis.
- Of those who have tried cannabis, 1 in 10 develop some form of psychological dependence syndrome.
- Significant numbers are reporting experience with more than one illegal drug – 45% of 'ever-users' have tried two or more.
- Many people stop taking drugs of their own volition – in one survey, of the 32% of 17–18 year olds who had tried an illegal drug, 10% no longer took them.

You can look at recent research projects and preliminary conclusions for the treatment or management of drug abuse on the website 'drugs abuse research initiative'.[4]

Case study 5.1

You call in Jo Bother, a 15 year old. Mr and Mrs Bother come in, but no son. They explain that they are worried about his recent change in behaviour. They have only recently discovered at a parents' evening that his school work has deteriorated and he has been missing school. He is often 'at a mate's house' in the evenings and is sullen and uncommunicative. He ignores his new clothes, wearing old scruffy ones and rarely seems to wash. When you ask what they are worried about, they look at each other and then say 'drugs'. They say that they feel very ignorant about drug use and don't know what to look out for, or whether they just have a difficult teenager.

What issues you should cover

Adolescence is a time for trying new things. Teenagers use drugs for many reasons, including curiosity, because it feels good, to reduce stress, to feel grown up or to fit in. It is difficult to know who will experiment and stop and who will develop serious problems. Unfortunately, teenagers often don't see the link between their actions today and the consequences tomorrow. They also have a tendency to feel indestructible and immune to the problems that others experience. Teenagers at risk of developing serious alcohol and drug problems include those who:

- have a family history of substance abuse
- are depressed
- have low self-esteem
- feel like they don't fit in or are out of the mainstream
- have poor or no job prospects
- are looked after in care homes or foster homes
- live in poverty or have a parent in prison.

Possible signs of illegal drug use may include:

- fatigue, repeated health complaints, red and glazed eyes, and a persistent cough
- personality change, sudden mood changes, irritability, irresponsible behaviour, low self-esteem, poor judgement, depression, and a general lack of interest
- starting arguments, breaking rules, or withdrawing from the family
- decreased interest, negative attitude, a drop in grades at school, many absences, truancy, and discipline problems
- new friends who are less interested in standard home and school activities; problems with the law, and changes to less conventional styles in dress and music
- poor time-keeping, poor work record or losing their job.

All of these may also be present in teenagers who are not using illegal drugs. They are little help in deciding whether Jo Bother is actually using illegal drugs, or just being a moody and rebellious teenager. His parents will actually have to try and confront the issue themselves.

Involving friends, teenagers of a similar age or siblings in talking to an adolescent may be helpful. Giving a teenager website contacts may be one way of letting them see for themselves what others think about drug taking and the dangers that they might be running.[5] Parents, like Mr and Mrs Bother, often feel pushed away and ignored but can offer support and understanding that rebellion and experimentation are normal teenage activities – but that they wish to offer some protection against harmful activities.[6] If a teenager is distressed and can be offered therapy or support, he or she can look at issues of motivation, build skills to resist drug use, replace drug-using activities with constructive and rewarding behaviours, and improve problem-solving skills. Behavioural therapy also facilitates interpersonal relationships and the teenager's ability to function in the home and community. Many schools have student counsellors and pastoral staff members who can offer support to teenagers who are going through this difficult transition, whether or not drug use is involved. Some young people will value help from inside the family, from their parents, or from siblings or other relatives. Confiding their feelings to an aunt, uncle or grandparent can sometimes be easier than to their own parents. It can be very difficult for parents or others close to the teenager to resist coming across as parental and authoritarian while avoiding condoning anti-social or harmful behaviour. Other young people want to talk only to other young people and value support from older peers or siblings, but this can place a big strain on people with limited emotional maturity themselves.

Collecting data to demonstrate your learning, competence, performance and standards of service delivery

Example cycle of evidence 5.1

- Focus: clinical care
- Other relevant foci: working with colleagues; relationships with patients

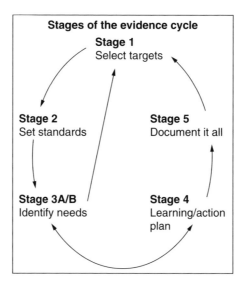

> **Case study 5.2**
>
> Dr New returned from working in New Zealand to join a general practice as a partner seven months ago. Shortly after he started work, Dr New saw Truly Stone and had referred her for antenatal care. Now she is back, looking terrible, thin, unkempt and miserable. Truly tells him that she had a premature labour and a stillbirth. She and her partner have been injecting heroin, but she wants to come off it and try for another baby, as that's what they really want. She blames Dr New for not telling her about the risks to her pregnancy when she first attended.

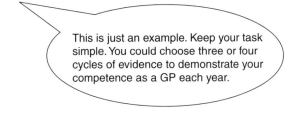

This is just an example. Keep your task simple. You could choose three or four cycles of evidence to demonstrate your competence as a GP each year.

Stage 1: Select your aspirations for good practice

The excellent GP:

- refers appropriately to other services
- communicates with colleagues
- gives patients appropriate information about their medical problems or condition.

Stage 2: Set the standards for your outcomes

Outcomes might include:

- the way learning is applied
- a learnt skill
- a protocol
- a strategy that is implemented
- meeting recommended standards.

- The referral pathways for patients with drug abuse problems are easily accessible to health professionals in the primary care team.

- There are clear communication procedures between midwives and the rest of the primary care team.
- The practice has written information to give to patients about drug misuse.

Stage 3A: Identify your learning needs

- Carry out with other practice staff a significant event audit looking for any preventive steps to avoid harm that could have been taken for Truly Stone.
- Record in your own reflective diary trends or comments relating to problems or issues of drug misuse in patients. This might be to do with the availability of services or about attitudes or lack of knowledge or skills in consultations with you, other health professionals and staff.
- Do a notes review to audit how often, or if, you discuss drug abuse in young women who consult you in early pregnancy, as well as discussing smoking, alcohol use and current prescribed or purchased medication.

Stage 3B: Identify your service needs

> Any of the needs assessment exercises in 3A may also reveal service needs.

- Audit the accessibility of drug abuse services.
- Obtain the local statistics about the scale of the problem of drug abuse in pregnancy.
- Observe the pathway of care received by a patient referred for antenatal care and the methods of communication of special risks to the midwives.
- Ask the person responsible for patient information literature in your practice to collect up and review all the information available on illegal drugs for accuracy and availability.

Stage 4: Make and carry out a learning and action plan

- Read about drug use in pregnancy.[7] Reflect how to use this knowledge in your consultations with young women in early pregnancy, or presenting for pregnancy advice.
- Read the patient literature on illegal drug use and assess its relevance and whether it is up to date. Make a list in a file on the practice computer of where it is available in the practice.
- Discuss at a practice meeting the communication with, and pathway for referral to, the community midwives.[8]
- Visit a practice in another area where there is a service for delivering appropriate care for pregnant women who have drug abuse problems.

- Discuss the significant event analysis at a practice meeting to which the midwives are invited, and decide on how to implement better communication and harm reduction for the future, bearing in mind the local scale of the problem.

Stage 5: Document your learning, competence, performance and standards of service delivery

- Document how you will use your increased knowledge in your consultations with young women in early pregnancy, or presenting for pregnancy advice.
- Keep a copy of the available patient literature on illegal drug use in a file on the computer.
- Record the outcome of the discussion at the practice meeting about the communication with, and pathway for referral to, the midwives.
- Record your observations following your visit to a practice where there is a service for delivering appropriate care for pregnant women who have drug abuse problems.
- Record the outcome of the discussion of the significant event analysis and how harm reduction will be implemented.

Case study 5.2 continued

The significant event audit shows that Truly Stone had been seen at the end of a surgery session that was running late. The member of staff who normally did the paperwork for registering patients for antenatal care had gone home. Truly had not returned for several weeks to complete the process, and often defaulted from her antenatal care. There were communication gaps between the general medical services provided for Truly and the midwives, which they both agreed to change. Truly had not attended the drug management scheme, as it was in a town 17 miles away. The practice team identified that there were an increasing number of young people at risk of harm from drug misuse. Dr New agreed to find out more about whether the practice could provide a better service for young people in the local area who were misusing drugs.

Example cycle of evidence 5.2

- Focus: teaching and training
- Other relevant focus: working with colleagues

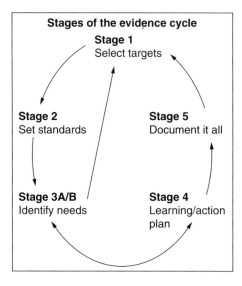

Stages of the evidence cycle

Stage 1
Select targets

Stage 2
Set standards

Stage 5
Document it all

Stage 3A/B
Identify needs

Stage 4
Learning/action
plan

Case study 5.3

Dr Green was doing her first six months of her GP registrar post and told you, as her trainer, about the patient she saw the day before. Her last patient of the day, Mr Charm, told her that he had moved to the area to get away from the stresses of living in London. Mr Charm had obtained a post as a media studies lecturer in the nearby city, but had decided to live in the country outside the market town where the practice is situated. He had rented accommodation in a holiday cottage and they had had a pleasant chat about his new rural lifestyle. He explained that he had some problems with drugs and was currently on diazepam as he learns to cope without. She said that she was taken aback when he asked for a month's supply of 40 mg a day. She explained that she would have to ask one of the partners, as she thought there was a practice policy about this. She rang the trainer's room, but there was no reply. Mr Charm had looked pointedly at his watch and said that he was right out of diazepam, as he could not get an appointment earlier. The chemist would have shut soon. She was swayed by his courtesy and friendliness, and agreed to write a prescription, arranging to see him again in two weeks.

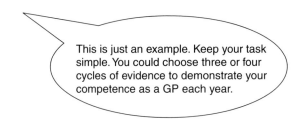

This is just an example. Keep your task simple. You could choose three or four cycles of evidence to demonstrate your competence as a GP each year.

Stage 1: Select your aspirations for good practice

The excellent GP:

- resists the temptation to appear superior by denigrating the care patients have received from others
- recognises and works within the limits of his/her competence and refers to another practitioner when indicated
- makes an adequate assessment of the patient's condition.

Stage 2: Set the standards for your outcomes

Outcomes might include:

- the way learning is applied
- a learnt skill
- a protocol
- a strategy that is implemented
- meeting recommended standards.

- Show that the trainer is accessible and able to give guidance when the GP registrar requires assistance.
- Develop the skills, attitudes and practices of a competent teacher.
- Demonstrate and communicate best practice in providing clinical care for people with drug problems.

Stage 3A: Identify your learning needs

- Assess your teaching and training skills e.g. by an external assessment organised as part of an external course.
- Check that your knowledge and skills about best practice in providing clinical care for people with drug problems is up to date and correct.
- Reflect on how best to help the GP registrar improve her consultation skills so that she is able to view manipulative patients more objectively.

Stage 3B: Identify your service needs

Any of the needs assessment exercises in 3A may also reveal service needs.

- Identify how the GP registrar can obtain support and advice during consultations when necessary.
- Find out about provision for support for Mr Charm and other similar patients.
- Establish how Dr Green could have contacted Mr Charm's previous GP or specialist.
- Identify with the practice team if the GP registrar is an appropriate person to be arranging the medical care for a new patient.

Stage 4: Make and carry out a learning and action plan

- Attend an external course to improve your teaching and training skills.
- Discuss the supervision needs of the GP registrar at a practice meeting and draw up a timetable of who is available and when.
- You and the practice secretary explore various sources of help for people abusing drugs and for those who wish to stop, and make a resource file for the practice computer system.
- Read about drug users, types of drugs and procedures for coming off drugs, making notes for a discussion with the GP registrar.
- Discuss at a trainers' meeting the best ways of improving the consultation skills of registrars.

Stage 5: Document your learning, competence, performance and standards of service delivery

- Record your attendance and the outcome of your evaluation at the external course to improve your teaching and training skills.
- Keep a copy of the timetable of who is available and when for the supervision needs of the GP registrar.
- Include a copy of the resource file for the practice computer system about the various sources of help for people abusing drugs and for those who wish to stop.
- Keep a copy of your notes of the discussion with the GP registrar about drug users, types of drugs and procedures for coming off drugs.
- Record the methods you employed for improving the consultation skills of the GP registrar.

Case study 5.3 continued

Dr Green was able to contact the unit where Mr Charm was seen before he moved. A copy of his management plan was faxed to the practice. You and Dr Green found out where he could be offered support for his withdrawal more locally. When Dr Green saw Mr Charm again, she was able to offer more practical help, and discuss his management plan with him. Dr Green practised with some case scenarios and discussed her interactions with patients with you, so that she becomes better able to recognise when she might be being manipulated. The contact list for help and advice for the GP registrar worked well until people went on holiday, and you had to discuss it again at another practice meeting.

References

1   Parliamentary Office of Science and Technology (1996) *Common Illegal Drugs and Their Effects – cannabis, ecstasy, amphetamines and LSD* is available from the Parliamentary Office of Science and Technology (POST), 7 Millbank, London SW1P 3JA (Tel: +44 (0)20 7219 2840).

2   Department of Health Annual report on the UK drug situation 2001. www.dh.gov.uk/assetRoot/04/03/44/29/04034429.pdf

3   www.homeoffice.gov.uk/rds/pdfs/hors224.pdf

4   www.mdx.ac.uk/www/drugsmisuse/execsummary.html

5   www.teenagehealthfreak.org/homepage/index.asp

6   Families Anonymous: for relatives and friends concerned about the use of drugs or related behavioural problems. Helpline +44 (0)845 1200 660; www.famanon.org.uk/professionals.html

7   www.babycentre.co.uk/refcap/541318.html

8   www.dh.gov.uk/PolicyAndGuidance/ResearchAndDevelopment/ResearchAndDevelopmentAZ/MotherAndChildHealth/MotherAndChildHealthArticle/fs/en?CONTENT_ID=4016310&chk=DU0Fst

6

Alcohol problems

Alcohol misuse is a major public health concern and has a huge impact on the economy, both in relation to healthcare costs and lost productivity at work.[1] General practice is ideally suited to help both identify and treat patients with alcohol misuse problems, having the dual advantage of seeing large numbers of patients and being able to provide them with opportunistic health promotion.[2] GPs see on average 360 patients each year who are misusing alcohol. Six out of ten GPs intervene with seven or fewer of these patients. At a conservative estimate, this suggests a 'failure to diagnose and failure to treat' six million people.

Case study 6.1

Ms Quaff is a 39-year-old professional woman who attends your surgery complaining of severe anxiety. You have not seen her before even though she has been registered with the surgery for three years. You find out that she is the human resources director of a large retail firm, travels a great deal and is barely at home for more than three consecutive days. She feels anxious every morning and finds that the symptoms persist throughout the day. She finds it difficult to sleep at night, not helped by her frequent travelling across time zones. She begins to cry and what emerges is that she may be drinking too much. You ask her more and find out that she consumes on average five 'small' gins most evenings and around a bottle of wine with her meal every evening.

What issues you should cover

Around 4% of the adult population are 'harmful drinkers' causing imminent risk to health. A further 23% are described as 'hazardous' drinkers, at increasing risk of health and injury, a considerable 8.8 million people in England (*see* Box 6.1 for definitions).

Box 6.1:   Definitions of alcohol abuse

- *Hazardous drinking*: consuming 22–50 units a week for men and 15–35 units a week for women, and carries increasing risk to health.
- *Harmful drinking*: consuming more than 50 units a week for men and 35 units a week for women and causing imminent risk to health.
- *Binge drinking*: men regularly drinking 10 or more units in a single session, and women regularly drinking 7 or more units in a single session. This is more than double the daily sensible drinking benchmark.
- *Alcohol dependence* (the term used in preference to 'alcoholism'): periodic or chronic intoxication, uncontrolled craving, tolerance resulting in dose increase and dependence on drinking alcohol.

Hazardous drinkers are unlikely to seek treatment for their drinking, and usually they do not actually need treatment as such. What they do need is early identification and early intervention, based on proven clinical techniques.

Presentation[3]

Patients who abuse alcohol may present in primary care with:

- depressed mood or failed treatment for depression
- nervousness
- insomnia
- physical complications such as stomach ulcer, gastritis, liver disease, hypertension
- accidents or injuries due to alcohol misuse
- poor memory or concentration
- evidence of self-neglect such as poor hygiene
- legal or social problems such as marital problems, domestic violence, child abuse or neglect, absence from work
- signs of withdrawal from alcohol: sweating, tremors, morning sickness, hallucinations, seizures
- a request for help: family members because the patient who is abusing alcohol denies problem, or the person themself presents for help or advice.

History taking

Ms Quaff is obviously drinking a lot of alcohol. It is important to try and determine the extent that her drinking has become a problem, that is, falling into the 'problem drinking' category, and how dependent she is. Complete the alcohol history, obtaining as accurate an account as possible of how much, when and in what circumstances she drinks. So, for example, when she says small gin, is this a home measure, which is often much more than a single pub measure, or is it the small bottle (equivalent to a double measure) often sold or given free in planes? Does she drink a bottle of wine every night in addition to the five gins? If one unit is a single measure of spirit, half a pint of normal strength lager or a small glass of wine (a bottle has about five glasses) then she is drinking between 10 and 15 units per day or 70–105 units per week, well above the recommended level for women (*see* Figure 6.1).

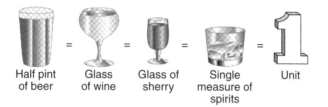

Figure 6.1:   Units contained in different drinks.

Try and find out how long Ms Quaff has been following this pattern. Look especially for the following:[3]

- stereotyped drinking pattern (same drink, same time)
- craving
- early morning drinking
- drinking to offset uncomfortable withdrawal symptoms such as 'the shakes'
- loss of control, often associated with blackouts
- tolerance: able to drink large quantities, rapidly developing even after a period of abstinence
- withdrawal symptoms, such as early morning retching, headache, sweating, shakes (these symptoms are often misinterpreted as anxiety).

Complications of alcohol use[4]

The complications of excess alcohol use affect every organ within the body. With Ms Quaff, focus on her psychological issues, such as depression, anxiety and panic attacks. Discuss the possible hazards of hypertension, menstrual disorders, gastritis, etc (*see* Table 6.1). Investigations may reveal abnormal liver function tests.

Table 6.1:   Estimates of proportion of death attributable to alcohol from various conditions in England and Wales[5]

Cause of death	*Percentage of deaths attributable to alcohol*
Cancer of the oesophagus	14–75
Cancer of the liver	15–29
Cancer of the female breast	3–4
Hypertension	5–11
Chronic pancreatitis	60–84
Acute pancreatitis	24–35
Falls	23–35
Drowning	30–38
Fire injuries	38–45
Suicide	27–41
Assault	27–47

Investigations

The three most commonly identified, and indeed most frequently used markers of alcohol misuse, are elevation of the erythrocyte mean corpuscular volume (MCV), and increases in serum aspartate aminotransferase (AST) and gamma glutamyl transpeptidase (GGT) levels. A number of other non-specific abnormalities such as hyperuricaemia and hypertriglyceridaemia may also be observed.

Case study 6.1 continued

Ms Quaff has been drinking heavily for seven years and has not had an alcohol-free day during this period. She realises that it is now getting out of hand but hadn't realised what a problem it actually was until she started talking to you. She wants to know what to do, whether to stop completely or to reduce her intake. Physical examination has shown that she is hypertensive. You arrange baseline blood investigations and arrange to see her again. In the meantime you suggest that she keeps an alcohol diary indicating when she drinks and the quantity, and give her some information (*see* Box 6.2) and a leaflet about 'women and alcohol'.[6]

Box 6.2:   Information about women and drinking alcohol
- More than 60% of all sexually transmitted infections (STIs) and unplanned pregnancies among students results from sexual encounters while one or more of the partners is drinking – interfering with adequate sexual decision making and practice of personal protection.
- More than 75% of 'acquaintance' rape and 60% of 'stranger' rape involve alcohol – either the perpetrator and/or the woman is drinking.
- The majority of domestic violence, including wife battering and child abuse, is associated with alcohol overuse.
- Women are more discrete at hiding their excessive alcohol intake and hence present for treatment much later than their male counterparts.
- Women are more likely to experience multiple dependence, especially on benzodiazepines and antidepressants.
- Treatment of alcohol abuse in women is more likely to include other co-morbid factors such as anorexia nervosa, depression, and anxiety.

Case study 6.1 continued

Ms Quaff returns two weeks later. Her liver function tests and full blood count are consistent with high alcohol use and her cholesterol is raised at 7.8 mmol/l.

Ms Quaff claims to only drink in the evenings, never to have had a drink in the morning and has not had blackouts or shakes. Her drink diary shows that she indeed does drink around 10 units of alcohol a night, though more if she is on business when it can rise to 20 units.

She has already begun to reduce her alcohol consumption, has talked to her bosses and asked to be transferred to a different section in the organisation, one that doesn't require as much travel. She was very grateful to you for un-covering her high alcohol consumption – something she had been worrying about for some time but was too ashamed to admit. She didn't realise how much damage it was doing to her though, and that it may even be related to her high blood pressure and high cholesterol.

Giving advice

Ms Quaff is drinking excessively but may not be dependent. You suggest that though her drinking is excessive, controlled drinking may be a realistic option. Tactics include:

- drinking modestly, no more than two standard drinks per day, with one or two alcohol-free days a week

- spacing drinks with non-alcoholic beverages or low-alcohol drinks
- eating before drinking and eating when drinking
- quenching thirst on water or soft drinks
- avoiding joining in with 'rounds'.

Abstinence is recommended if there is established alcohol dependence, marked physical damage, or when controlled drinking has failed.

Brief and minimal interventions[7]

You have already started intervening just by taking a history and listening to her worries. Research has shown that spending even a few minutes with a patient, offering advice on reducing consumption and motivating in a non-judgemental fashion, can bring about change.[8] Interventions can be from a few minutes to several half-hour sessions; the term 'minimal brief interventions' is used to describe sessions of up to five minutes provided by a GP.

A meta-analysis found that excessive drinkers who received brief intervention were twice as likely to moderate their drinking when compared to excessive drinkers who did not receive any intervention.[9] 'Brief intervention' is generally restricted to four or fewer sessions, each session lasting from a few minutes to one hour, and is designed to be conducted by health professionals who do not specialise in addictions treatment. It is most often used with patients who are not alcohol dependent, and its goal may be to moderate drinking rather than achieve abstinence. Research indicates that brief intervention for alcohol problems is more effective than no intervention and is often as effective as more extensive intervention.[10]

The key ingredients of brief interventions are summarised by the acronym FRAMES:[7]

> **F**eedback
> **R**esponsibility
> **A**dvice
> **M**enu of strategies
> **E**mpathy
> **S**elf-efficacy.

Goal setting, follow-up, and timing have also been identified as important to the effectiveness of brief intervention.

Case study 6.1 continued

You see Ms Quaff fortnightly for the next six weeks and you learn that her father was an alcoholic. Ms Quaff finds it hard to control her drinking. She realises that she had been colluding with herself for years and that her drinking had caused her many problems.

She drops into your surgery about six months later. She has lost two stone in weight, looks 10 years younger and has changed her job. She has decided that she didn't trust herself to control her drinking and has actually abstained completely. Her blood pressure is now normal and you offer to repeat her blood tests for her.

Collecting data to demonstrate your learning, competence, performance and standards of service delivery

Example cycle of evidence 6.1

- Focus: management of alcohol misuse
- Other relevant foci: prescribing interactions; refusal of tests

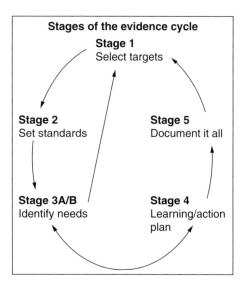

Stages of the evidence cycle

Stage 1
Select targets

Stage 2
Set standards

Stage 5
Document it all

Stage 3A/B
Identify needs

Stage 4
Learning/action plan

Case study 6.2

Ms Barr has returned to see you about her continuing depression. This is her second consultation, one month after being started on an antidepressant drug. Another GP had started her on treatment then and had noted in her records that she smelt of alcohol at the morning appointment, and requested blood tests to investigate (full blood count including MCV and liver function tests). Her blood results are not back and you find that she did not actually arrange for her blood to be taken. 'What was the point – I know I am drinking too much, I don't need any tests to tell me that!' Ms Barr feels a little better for taking her antidepressants, she is sleeping longer in the morning and is less weepy but still basically depressed. She asks you to examine her swollen and cut knees while she is there – a result of a fall down some stairs. You try to discuss exactly how much alcohol she is drinking and to find out how dependent she is on alcohol, e.g. by asking the CAGE questions.[11] You wonder how to proceed with someone who does not want to accept help for her admitted problem with alcohol and if it is safe to continue the antidepressant drug without knowing her liver function.

> This is just an example. Keep your task simple. You could choose three or four cycles of evidence to demonstrate your competence as a GP each year.

Stage 1: Select your aspirations for good practice

The excellent GP:

- respects the right of patients to refuse treatments or tests
- is up to date with developments in clinical practice
- chooses specialists to meet the needs of individual patients.

Stage 2: Set the standards for your outcomes

Outcomes might include:

- the way learning is applied
- a learnt skill
- a protocol
- a strategy that is implemented
- meeting recommended standards.

- Have an agreed practice protocol describing the team management of alcohol misuse.
- Become the clinical lead in the practice for patients who misuse alcohol.

Stage 3A: Identify your learning needs

- Chat on the phone with the community psychiatric nurse (CPN) who specialises in helping patients who misuse alcohol, and ask his advice about any techniques for helping people who are not motivated to change. Find out what you 'do not know you do not know'.
- Think about what you know about which drugs are contraindicated where alcohol is known to be misused or liver function is deranged. Look up the contraindications to prescribing a range of antidepressant drugs in the *British National Formulary* to check your knowledge.[1 2]
- Talk to other colleagues in the practice about their approach when patients refuse tests or treatment. Find out if you (and they) have learning needs about the legal position.
- Make a list of the symptoms or signs commonly encountered in patients who are misusing alcohol. Compare your list with the World Health Organization document.[3]

Stage 3B: Identify your service needs

> Any of the needs assessment exercises in 3A may also reveal service needs.

- Audit the number of referrals from the practice in the last 12 months of patients who misuse alcohol (and other substances) to CPNs or other specialists in the community or in secondary care. How does your referral pattern compare with that of other practices? Could a low referral rate indicate that your practice team is detecting few patients who are abusing alcohol? Alternatively a low referral rate might be because you and colleagues are good at managing such cases in the practice.
- Ask your CPN colleague what services are available for people misusing alcohol for you to refer to or patients to self-refer – are you aware of them all?
- Do you know what you can do to optimise the referral? Find out the extent and type of information about the patient that will help to prioritise referrals. You could discuss this with the CPN to find out if there are other gaps in what you are doing as a practice team.

Stage 4: Make and carry out a learning and action plan

- Read about the management of patients who abuse alcohol. Locate national or local guidelines on the diagnosis and management of alcohol misuse in primary care.
- Attend a health promotion workshop that covers training in motivating patients to change adverse lifestyle habits.
- After obtaining the patient's informed consent, sit in on a consultation of your CPN or psychiatrist specialising in alcohol misuse, with a patient you have referred for help. Watch their approach and learn what else you might have been able to do in your consultation with the patient. Keep a close watch on the patient's progress and outcomes of successive appointments with the specialist.
- Draw up a practice protocol based on what you have learnt about approach and services from undertaking the learning and service needs assessments. Adapt the national or local guidelines to the setting of your practice.
- Hold an in-house educational session with other GPs and nurses plus the practice manager, to explain the protocol to the others in your practice team, and gain their ownership. Use the audit of referrals as a focus for any action that needs to be taken.

Stage 5: Document your learning, competence, performance and standards of service delivery

- Include a copy of the new practice protocol.
- Include an anonymised copy of the audit of referrals, the conclusion and any action taken.
- Keep a copy of your notes of the in-house educational session. Comment on the barriers and other issues coming out of the discussion about the protocol, and what you will do as a team to make the protocol work.
- Include a copy of literature for patients to explain how they can get help for problems with alcohol.

Case study 6.2 continued

You are able to continue Ms Barr's antidepressant drug, which does not appear to be contraindicated. Two appointments later, Ms Barr is starting to talk to you about her drinking habits. She agrees that she wants to do something about it and does go to the nurse for her blood tests. Ms Barr also agrees she will go and see a specialist CPN about her addiction to alcohol but she does not attend that appointment.

Example cycle of evidence 6.2

- Focus: managing suspicions of child abuse
- Other relevant foci: deciding to breach patient confidentiality; relationships with patients; teamworking

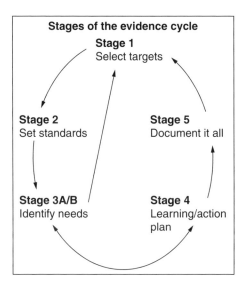

Stages of the evidence cycle

Stage 1
Select targets

Stage 2
Set standards

Stage 5
Document it all

Stage 3A/B
Identify needs

Stage 4
Learning/action plan

Case study 6.3

Mrs Brunt is nursing a swollen eye when she brings in one of her two little girls, Pat. After examining Pat's eczema and printing off a prescription, you ask Mrs Brunt about her eye. It all comes pouring out – her husband's occasional violence after he has had too much to drink (as happened last week), their fear, their debts. Mrs Brunt has almost made up her mind to leave her husband and take the girls with her. She tells you her plans but they seem rather vague. You enquire further about whether their father is ever violent towards the girls and, although Mrs Brunt denies it, you have the gut feeling from the reactions of both Mrs Brunt and Pat that the girls are at risk.

This is just an example. Keep your task simple. You could choose three or four cycles of evidence to demonstrate your competence as a GP each year.

Stage 1: Select your aspirations for good practice

The excellent GP:

- acts promptly where child protection is an issue
- makes appropriate judgements about patients who need referral
- respects the patient's right to confidentiality and provides information to colleagues in a manner appropriate to their level of involvement in the patient's care.

Stage 2: Set the standards for your outcomes

> Outcomes might include:
>
> - the way learning is applied
> - a learnt skill
> - a protocol
> - a strategy that is implemented
> - meeting recommended standards.

- Know when it is good practice to breach patient confidentiality and how to do it.
- Take action in line with local referral protocol and procedures for child protection.

Stage 3A: Identify your learning needs

- Consider what you should do when you have vague suspicions that a child may be at risk of domestic violence or other abuse. Discuss the action you might take with the child protection lead in your PCO.
- Obtain local protocol and national guidance for child protection and compare what you think you should do with what the protocol states.[13]
- Ring the local medical committee or PCO officer to compare what you think and what they recommend about you passing on confidential information to social services (about your suspicions of violence towards Pat Brunt and her sister from their drunken father when you have no evidence).

Stage 3B: Identify your service needs

> Any of the needs assessment exercises in 3A may also reveal service needs.

- Undertake a significant event audit of any incident involving child abuse. Analyse with colleagues whether you and others acted in accordance with best practice protocols or local guidelines.
- Look at the practice protocol about confidentiality and identify the circumstances in which confidential information can be relayed to others without the patient's explicit consent. Compare it with official guidance from your medical defence society or the Department of Health.[14]
- Audit the outcomes of five patients whom you have coded as abusing alcohol. Reflecting on their cases, could more be done in the practice to proactively engage patients in treatment earlier? Could more or different care be provided once those patients have admitted their problems with alcohol?
- If Mr Brunt is registered with the practice, look at his medical records. Search to see if he has an entry about a problem with alcohol and, if so, could the practice team do more? If there is no record of his problem with alcohol, log the information given by his wife and consider if, in retrospect, he has consulted with symptoms and signs that may be attributable to his reported alcohol problem. This might indicate that you or others need to learn to be more alert to the ways in which those who abuse alcohol may present.

Stage 4: Make and carry out a learning and action plan

- Discussions with colleagues (as in Stage 3) will be part of the learning and action plan.
- Reading up on the protocols and guidance described in Stage 3 will form part of your learning plan.
- Attend a workshop on alcoholism.
- Run two in-house educational sessions with your practice team to discuss and formulate action following the results of the significant event analysis (child protection) and audit (patients with problems with alcohol) as described in Stage 3.

Stage 5: Document your learning, competence, performance and standards of service delivery

- Include a reference to the local child protection protocol.
- Include a copy of the booklet describing action professionals should take to safeguard children.[13]
- Record the action plans from the in-house educational discussions of audits, with the repeat audits done or planned for six months later.
- Include an audit of the next case of suspected or proven child abuse occurring in the practice and compare the management with best practice (against the local protocol or national guidance).

Case study 6.3 continued

You ask the practice nurse to take Pat to play with a box of toys for a few minutes while you talk privately with her mother. You express your fears about the possibility of Mr Brunt being violent with the children, which she again denies. You discuss your fears with colleagues in the practice and they urge you to contact social services to talk over your concerns, for which you have little evidence. The duty social worker assures you that you have taken the right action and they will investigate the circumstances. Your suspicions prove to be correct, and Pat's older sister does have bruises too from when her Dad lashed out at her the previous week.

The father is not a patient at the practice, so you cannot offer him help with his drinking problem. From what you learn in this exercise, you are much clearer about what action you could have taken.

Example cycle of evidence 6.3

- Focus: relationships with patients
- Other relevant foci: clinical care; health promotion; teaching

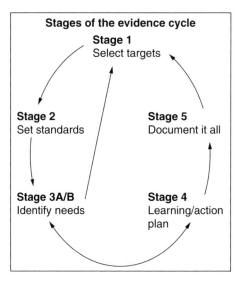

Stages of the evidence cycle

Stage 1
Select targets

Stage 2
Set standards

Stage 5
Document it all

Stage 3A/B
Identify needs

Stage 4
Learning/action plan

Case study 6.4

Rocky comes to see you in the university vacation. He is consulting you because of his morning sickness, sweating and, most of all, the tremor of his hands that makes working on the computer keyboard difficult. He is in his third year at university and staying at his parents' home – out in the sticks. You ask him to tell you more about himself. His face lights up as he tells you about the 'wicked' time he has at uni with his mates, out clubbing, doing some lectures but missing others. He cannot wait to get back to Uni as he rarely goes out at night when staying at his parents' home, being stuck out in the countryside without transport.

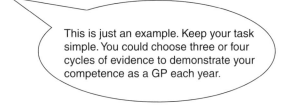

This is just an example. Keep your task simple. You could choose three or four cycles of evidence to demonstrate your competence as a GP each year.

Stage 1: Select your aspirations for good practice

The excellent GP:

- uses clear language appropriate for the patient
- uses investigations when they will help the management of the condition
- promotes a healthy lifestyle to all patients.

Stage 2: Set the standards for your outcomes

Outcomes might include:

- the way learning is applied
- a learnt skill
- a protocol
- a strategy that is implemented
- meeting recommended standards.

- Be able to motivate patients to pursue healthy lifestyles.

Stage 3A: Identify your learning needs

- Seek feedback from patients whom you have advised about their unhealthy lifestyles (poor or fatty diet, lack of exercise, smoking, excessive alcohol). Focus on the clarity of information you gave or way of giving it (your teaching skills).
- Seek feedback from colleagues about your ability to motivate patients with unhealthy lifestyles. Ask them to record their impressions when they have seen the same patients on subsequent occasions.
- Undertake an audit of 10 consecutive patients whom you have advised to stop smoking, lose weight, take up exercise, cut down or stop drinking alcohol. Follow them over time to see the results of your (and others') advice giving, by reviewing their notes one year later or asking them directly 6–12 months later when they consult you for the same or different conditions.

Stage 3B: Identify your service needs

> Any of the needs assessment exercises in 3A may also reveal service needs.

- Review all the literature that exists in the practice for advising patients who abuse alcohol or have a drinking problem. Is it current, clear, and relevant for different age groups? Ask patients of different age groups to 'proof read' them and comment on the way information is given.
- Undertake an audit of 50 patients whose age ranges from 16–24 years, to ascertain for how many you as a practice have recorded lifestyle details, including alcohol consumption. Also record what action or advice was given subsequently for any who were drinking more alcohol than is recommended for a healthy lifestyle.
- Draw up a patient pathway for a person like Rocky. Start from the first consultation with an alcohol-related symptom or sign and what investigations, treatment, advice should be offered. Discuss the pathway as a practice team to add in other alternative approaches that colleagues take and review how much similarity there is between individual team members.

Stage 4: Make and carry out a learning and action plan

- Attend a seminar run by health promotion to learn more about motivating patients. Establish how to maximise your impact if they are either not contemplating or are contemplating changing their lifestyles.
- Sit in on sessions with a colleague who has a good track record in motivating others to change their lifestyle e.g. in a structured smoking

cessation session, and learn what you can apply in the approaches you take to patients.
- Invite that expert colleague to critique your approach in a follow-up session with a patient you are trying to motivate to change their lifestyle (e.g. with the patient's permission for sitting in, or from an audio tape), and discuss your performance together.
- Run a focus group of young people to discuss the patient literature and how the practice might improve services, especially to help them attain healthy lifestyles. Involve others who might help develop improved services e.g. from a local leisure centre, youth club, etc.
- Write a protocol for yourself and the practice team on helping patients to attain a healthy lifestyle, including when liver function tests, full blood count and fasting lipids should be undertaken.

Stage 5: Document your learning, competence, performance and standards of service delivery

- Keep a copy of the practice protocol with the indications for blood tests and the action needed.
- Keep a copy of the audit and action and learning undertaken as a result.
- Keep the revised practice literature and links to leisure and youth services following the focus group meeting.
- Make a record of your reflections on what you have learnt about motivation techniques, from sitting in and the follow-up discussions with your expert colleague.
- Repeat the audit of 10 consecutive patients to demonstrate your improved skills in motivating people to switch to healthier lifestyles.

Case study 6.4 continued

Rocky is surprised and shocked that you think he is exhibiting symptoms of withdrawal from alcohol, as he had never considered it. He does not want to talk about it and rushes off. You see him again when he consults about his acne, six months later when he has finished his degree and moved back to the local area, in a flat with his friends. He tells you that he has really thought through how much alcohol he was drinking and realises that you were probably right. Since then he has not drunk alcohol when on his own – it was automatic before to have cans stashed around his bedroom. He has gone out less with his mates and although he still binges on alcohol at times, it is less often and he is gradually cutting down.

References

1 UK Alcohol Forum (1997) *Guidelines for the Management of Alcohol Problems in Primary Care and General Psychiatry.* Tangent Medical Education, London.

2 McAvoy BR (2000) Alcohol education for general practitioners in the United Kingdom – a window of opportunity? *Alcohol and Alcoholism.* **35:** 225–9.

3 Babor TF, Higgins-Biddle JC, Saunders JB and Monteiro MG (2001) *The Alcohol Use Disorders Identification Test. World Health Organization,* Geneva. http://whqlibdoc.who.int/hq/2001/WHO_MSD_MSB_01.6a.pdf

4 Royal College of Physicians (1987) *A Great and Growing Evil – the medical consequences of alcohol abuse.* Royal College of Physicians, London.

5 Greenfield TK (2001) Individual risk of alcohol related disease and problems. In: Heather N, Peters TJ and Stockwell T (eds) *International Handbook of Alcohol Dependence and Problems.* Wiley, London. www.dfc.unifi.it/sia/alcohoandhealth.pdf

6 www.acad.org.uk/04.html

7 Bien TH, Miller WR and Tonigan JS (1993) Brief interventions for alcohol problems: a review. *Addiction.* **88:** 315–36.

8 Wallace PG and Haines AP (1984) General practitioner and health promotion: what patients think. *British Medical Journal.* **289:** 534–6.

9 Wilk AI, Jensen NM and Havighurst TC (1997) Meta-analysis of randomised controlled trials addressing brief interventions in heavy alcohol drinkers. *Journal of General Internal Medicine.* **12:** 274–83.

10 Edwards G, Orford J, Egert S *et al.* (1997) Alcoholism: a controlled trial of 'treatment' and 'advice'. *Journal of Studies on Alcohol.* **38:** 1004–31.

11 http://www.netdoctor.co.uk/health_advice/facts/alcoholism.htm

12 Joint Formulary Committee (2003) *British National Formulary.* British Medical Association and Royal Pharmaceutical Society of Great Britain, London. www.bnf.org

13 Department of Health (2003) What to do if you're worried a child is being abused. HMSO, London. www.dh.gov.uk/assetRoot/04/06/13/03/04061303.pdf

14 Department of Health (2003) *Confidentiality. NHS Code of Practice.* Department of Health, London.

Further reading

Managing the heavy drinker in primary care (2000) *Drug and Therapeutics Bulletin.* **3:** 60–4.

Ashworth M and Gerada C (1998) Addiction and dependence-alcohol. In: T Davies and TK Craig (eds) *ABC of Mental Health.* BMJ Publications, London.

Deehan A, Marshall EJ and Strang J (1998) Tackling alcohol misuse: opportunities and obstacles in primary care. *British Journal of General Practice.* **48:** 1779–82.

McAvoy BR (1997) Training general practitioners. *Alcohol and Alcoholism.* **32:** 9–12.

McAvoy BR, Kaner EF, Lock C *et al.* (1999) Our Healthier Nation – are general practitioners willing and able to deliver? A survey of attitudes to and involvement in health promotion and lifestyle counselling. *British Journal of General Practice.* **49:** 187–90.

Kaner EF, Heather N, Mc Avoy BR *et al.* (1999) Intervention for excessive alcohol consumption in primary health care: attitudes and practices of English general practitioners. *Alcohol and Alcoholism.* **34:** 559–66.

Fleeman ND (1997) Alcohol home detoxification: a literature review. *Alcohol and Alcoholism.* **32:** 649–56.

7

Common arthritis problems

Rheumatoid arthritis

This autoimmune disorder typically involves many joints and often many other body systems. Most patients have a fluctuating course that results in progressive joint destruction, deformity and disability. Inability or reduction of ability to do productive work causes economic loss to individuals and society. It affects about 0.5% of the population.[1] An easily assimilated reference book, such as the *ABC of Rheumatology*, will help to remind you of the salient features.[2] The prognosis after diagnosis is unpredictable. Some people experience flare-ups and remissions, others an unremitting progression. Over the years, joint deformities and functional impairment occur with structural damage to the joints. About half of those diagnosed will be disabled or unable to work after 10 years, and it shortens life expectancy.[3,4]

Case study 7.1

Mr Stone, a seed salesman aged 43 years, comes to see you. He tells you that he cannot work as his hands and feet are too painful. His metacarpo-phalangeal and finger joints are swollen. He says they were red but that has gone now. When you look at his feet, the appearance is similar but less marked. He has tenderness along the joint lines and winces when you palpate the joints. He has some other aches and pains but none as severe. He, and the previous doctor he saw two weeks ago, had assumed the joints were inflamed because he had been rebuilding a stone wall that had fallen into a stream on his property, standing in the cold water for long periods of time and lifting cold stones. He is sleeping badly as the pain wakes him and is poorly controlled by the ibuprofen and solpadeine that he is taking. He wants to know what you think it is and how long it will last.

What issues you should cover

Excluding urgent conditions

When presented with acute joint pain, your most important task is to ensure that you identify serious conditions that need urgent evaluation. There are three types of condition that you do not want to miss – malignancy, bone or joint sepsis, and major vessel or nerve damage, so look out for the 'red flags' that suggest that one or other of these conditions may be present (*see* Table 7.1). In addition, check for a history of serious trauma, which can result in fractures or unstable joints.[5]

Table 7.1: 'Red flags' requiring urgent action

Condition	Symptoms and signs
Sepsis	Hot swollen joint, fever, redness over a very tender bone or joint, general malaise, weight loss
Malignancy	General ill-health, malaise, weight loss, severe constant pain in bones, not affected by rest or exercise
Neurovascular damage	Burning pain radiating in a nerve or nerve root distribution, claudication, cold white extremities, sensory or motor loss

Assessment of disability and pain

It is important to find out what disability results from the condition. Lower limb problems may cause walking difficulties, and upper limb problems difficulty with reaching and dexterity. So good questions to ask are:

- *'Do you have any difficulty climbing stairs?'* (if a patient can climb stairs and steps, he or she can walk and get on buses).
- *'Do you have any difficulty washing or dressing yourself?'* (impairments of dexterity, reaching and personal care are common, and washing and dressing are among the most important tasks to be affected).

In addition, other impairments may make things much worse, so it is always worth asking about sensory problems, such as problems with sight or hearing, especially in older people.

Psychosocial factors are important. Pain and loss of ability to do previously achieved tasks is depressing, and causes anxiety and loss of self-esteem. This makes the pain more difficult to bear. Occupation may be important, as many common musculoskeletal problems are overuse injuries.

Case study 7.1 continued

You take a fuller history and rule out any 'red flags'. Mr Stone has prolonged morning stiffness and pain that gradually improves as he moves around. The pain is worse if he tries to grasp anything, and he is having difficulty writing and cutting up his food. He thought he had caught a chill working in the cold water as he felt a bit hot and cold, and generally unwell, but he had been well before starting on the wall. He rubs his eyes and says he thought he might have got a bit of stone dust in them, as they had been quite sore. He has not had any previous joint trouble and has had no rash, or skin condition, such as psoriasis. He has never had any trouble with having cold hands or feet that become red or purple and might suggest Raynaud's phenomenon. He takes no other medication.

Making the diagnosis

The history gives you a good idea of the type of musculoskeletal pathology present and whether the pain is inflammatory or mechanical in nature. Examination sorts out the anatomical source of the pain.[6]

The type of pain, where the pain is and what makes it better or worse gives you clues about what might cause it:

- prolonged morning stiffness in multiple painful joints and some improvement with exercise usually indicates an inflammatory rheumatic condition such as rheumatoid arthritis (RA). These symptoms may be accompanied by feeling ill, fever, weight loss, and signs and symptoms of involvement of other parts of the body such as dry eyes and mouth, rashes, red eyes, urethritis, adenopathy, oral ulcers, pleuritic chest pain, or Raynaud's phenomenon
- shorter morning stiffness with little or no pain at rest, with pain increasing during or after sustained exercise, suggests local mechanical problems (bursitis, tendonitis, sprains and strains) or osteoarthritis (OA), especially if there is no systemic illness
- pain from articular structures is usually worse on movement or weight bearing, and relieved by rest
- pain described as numbness, burning, shooting, or pins and needles is likely to be neurological, especially if its distribution is localised to a dermatome, peripheral nerve or a stocking-glove type
- claudication pain from arterial insufficiency occurs during use and is relieved by rest; lumbar spinal stenosis neurogenic pain presents with pain on walking that is relieved slowly by sitting or spinal flexion

- pain that is vaguely localised to a joint, but where the joint appears normal, can be due to referred pain or a bone lesion. Bone lesions often cause unceasing night pain.

Table 7.2 describes useful clinical features to distinguish between types of musculoskeletal pain.

Table 7.2:   Useful clinical features when evaluating a patient with musculoskeletal pain

	Periarticular problem	*OA or internal derangement*	*Inflammatory rheumatic disease*
Symptoms			
Morning stiffness	Usually absent	Local, short-lived	Severe and prolonged
Worst time	With use	With use	After prolonged inactivity
General ill-health	Not relevant	Not relevant	Often present
Locking or instability	Uncommon (only with tendonitis)	Implies a loose body, internal derangement, or weakness	Uncommon in early disease, may result from late joint damage
Symmetry	Uncommon	Occasional	Usual
Signs			
Tenderness	Focal, periarticular, (or tender points in fibromyalgia)	Over a single joint line	Over the joint line of all affected joints
Inflammation (fluid, warmth)	Occasionally over tendon or bursa	Absent or mild	Severe
Other systems involved	No	No	Sometimes

Regional musculoskeletal pain has three main causes:

- periarticular lesions such as tendonitis, bursitis and enthesopathies (problems at ligament or tendon insertions)
- mechanical problems of joints (such as internal derangements or osteoarthritis)
- inflammatory synovitis.

> **Case study 7.1 continued**
> Mr Stone's pattern of pain and the symmetrical nature of the inflammatory swelling of his joints suggest RA and you arrange some investigations. You change his non-steroidal anti-inflammatory drug (NSAID) warning him about the risks of indigestion and possibly even bleeding with higher stronger doses.

Treatment with non-steroidal anti-inflammatory drugs[7]

It is sensible to become familiar with the adverse profiles of a few NSAIDs. Include the selected drugs on your preferred drug list or practice formulary. You might divide them into traditional NSAIDs (like ibuprofen, naproxen, or diclofenac), cyclo-oxygenase-2 (Cox II)-preferential inhibitors, like meloxicam, and Cox II-selective inhibitors, like celecoxib. You are more likely to pick up an adverse effect quickly, and discontinue the drug, if you are aware of the possibility that the clinical picture is likely to have an iatrogenic cause. If all members of the practice team agree to use NSAIDs from a selected list, it will be much easier for all staff to be on the lookout for possible adverse effects.

Patients at high risk of gastrointestinal problems should receive anti-ulcer treatments with their NSAIDs. Misoprostol, omeprazole and ranitidine taken regularly have all been found to work better than a placebo in randomly controlled trials. However, the H_2 receptor antagonists that reduce acid secretion (ranitidine, cimetidine, famotizine, nizatidine) are not as effective as omeprazole (a proton pump inhibitor), or misoprostol (a prostaglandin analogue) for gastro-protection.[8] Some recent trials suggested that omeprazole may be most effective, but the studies were not strictly comparable with earlier trials.[8] Misoprostol causes more adverse effects – mainly abdominal pain and diarrhoea. Misoprostol may cause vaginal bleeding and should only be taken by women in their reproductive years if they are also taking adequate contraceptive precautions.

The presence of *Helicobacter pylori* is known to be associated with the development of peptic ulceration, and eradicating it often allows people to cease taking their anti-ulcer medication. A randomised trial of eradicating *H. pylori* in patients who needed to take NSAIDs suggests that this would be useful in reducing the risk of peptic ulcers.[9]

The more recently introduced Cox II inhibitors have become available with the hope of reducing the unwanted effects of NSAIDs on the gastrointestinal tract. They are as effective as other NSAIDs; dyspesia appears to occur as often, but the occurrence of ulcers by endoscopic examination was similar to an inert placebo medication.[9,10] Peripheral oedema, dizziness and skin rashes are still adverse reactions that may occur with the Cox II inhibitors as with other

NSAIDs. They are more expensive than most of the older NSAIDs and their use is limited by the presence in many arthritis sufferers of other medical conditions and interacting medications. Rofecoxib has been withdrawn from use because of the increased numbers of strokes and heart attacks after long-term use.[9]

Investigations

The diagnosis of early RA is made on the history and examination but may be confirmed by investigations. In the early stages of the disease, the results of investigations can be inconclusive or confusing. If after the history and your examination you conclude that the problem is a mechanical or extra-articular one, then investigations are unnecessary. Beware of doing investigations without thinking whether the results will alter your management. Abnormalities are often found in the absence of disease, especially as people grow older.

If you are unsure what tests are currently indicated, ask your laboratory for help, or consult an up-to-date reference guide.[11]

An erythrocyte sedimentation rate (ESR) or plasma viscosity (PV) test is non-specific, but useful if you suspect an infection, inflammation, or malignancy. A very high ESR suggests polymyalgia rheumatica, giant cell arteritis, or cancer. A C-reactive protein test is also raised in infection and inflammation and may be raised when the ESR is normal. It is more useful for monitoring response to disease-modifying drugs in RA. Complement is also used to monitor the disease activity. Single point measurements are of limited value as the various fractions are difficult to interpret.

Only request rheumatoid factor (RF) and/or anti-nuclear antibody (ANA) tests if you suspect a systemic rheumatoid disease. The higher the level of rheumatoid factor, the more likely that the diagnosis is rheumatoid arthritis (RA), but at least a quarter of patients with RA never have a raised level. Other inflammatory conditions such as systemic lupus erythematosus (SLE), or viral infections, may also show a positive RF. A high titre of anti-nuclear antibody makes SLE more likely, but false-positive tests often occur.

In patients with multisystem symptoms and signs, full blood count and biochemical screening to include liver and kidney function are usually done. Other tests can be performed for specific diagnostic possibilities (*see* Table 7.3). Synovial fluid needs examination in an acutely inflamed single joint, to rule out infection, and can be useful in sorting out other types of effusion or synovitis. For example, you might need to use it to differentiate pseudogout (in which calcium or crystal deposits fall out of the cartilage into the joint and cause synovial inflammation) from other causes of a red swollen knee.

Table 7.3:   Tests for other musculoskeletal causes for pain

Diagnosis suspected	Investigation
Viral arthritis	Hepatitis serology; Lyme or parvovirus, other viral studies
Myositis with muscle weakness	Creatinine phosphokinase; myositis-specific antibodies
Spondylitis	HLA-B27
Wegener's granulomatosis	Antineutrophil cytoplasmic antibody
Gout	Uric acid; may not be raised in acute attacks, check it between, or to monitor medication

HLA: human lymphocytic antigen

X-rays

Plain radiographs are not helpful for most patients who have acute or new symptoms and signs of RA, SLE, gout, mechanical back pain, tendonitis or bursitis. They may confirm the presence of OA, but can be normal in the early stages.

Imaging is indicated if you have a history of significant injury, when joint function is lost, when pain continues despite conservative management, or when there is a history of malignancy. A bone scan is useful if osteomyelitis or malignancy are suspected. Magnetic resonance imaging (MRI) should be reserved for patients in whom a specific abnormality is suspected.

Case study 7.1 continued

Mr Stone returns in a week with some relief from a change in NSAID and his sleep pattern has improved considerably. His ESR is raised, but his other tests are inconclusive with only a weakly positive RF.

You discuss early referral to a rheumatologist and explain about disease-modifying drugs and other treatments. Now he has less pain, you suggest ways he can keep active and move his joints to preserve function.

Referral

Refer early so that joint damage can be minimised by disease-modifying antirheumatic drugs (DMARDs). If you have a special interest in rheumatology, you may be starting your patient on these drugs yourself, or you may be able to refer more quickly to a practitioner with a special interest (PwSI) who can do this.[12] Shared care protocols for the management of people taking DMARDs are common. You must have monitoring systems for all patients on DMARDs and be prepared to show that they are effective (*see* Table 7.4).[13]

Table 7.4:   Guidelines for monitoring DMARDs

Drug	Maintenance dose	Toxicity	Tests
Hydroxy-chloroquine	200 mg twice daily	Rash (infrequent) diarrhoea, retinal toxicity (rare).	None unless symptoms present.
Sulphasalazine	1000 mg 2–3 times daily	Rash, myelosuppression (infrequent), GI intolerance.	Full blood count[a] (FBC) and liver function tests (LFTs) weekly for 1 month, monthly for 5 months, then every 6 months.
Methotrexate (toxic effects may be less with folic acid)	7.5–15 mg per week	GI symptoms, stomatitis, rash, alopecia, myelosuppression (infrequent), hepatoxicity, pulmonary toxicity (rare but serious).	FBC[a] monthly, LFT every 3 months.
Injectable gold salts	25–50 mg IM every 2–4 weeks	Rash, stomatitis, myelosuppression, thrombocytopenia, proteinuria.	FBC[a] and urinalysis weekly for 1 month, then monthly. If urine protein ++, send mid-stream urine (MSU). If MSU negative or protein +++, stop and refer.
Leflunomide	Loading dose 100 mg once daily for 3 days. Maintenance dose 10–20 mg daily.	Diarrhoea, rash, hair loss, hypertension, nausea, elevated liver enzymes.	Liver enzymes and blood pressure before treatment and periodically afterwards. FBC[a] before treatment and every 2 weeks for 6 months, then every 8 weeks.
Azathioprine	50–150 mg daily	Myelosuppression, hepatotoxicity (infrequent), early flu-like illness with fever, GI symptoms, elevated LFTs.	FBC[a] and LFT weekly for 1 month then monthly.
D-penicillamine	250–750 mg daily after initial very gradual increase in dose.	Rash, stomatitis, proteinuria, myelosuppression, autoimmune disease (rare but serious).	FBC[a] and urinalysis weekly for 2 months, then monthly.

[a] stop drug and refer if white blood cell count < 3.0 ($\times 10^9$/l), platelets < 120 ($\times 10^9$/l), or if LFTs are deteriorating

FBC: full blood count; LFT: liver function test; GI: gastrointestinal; IM: intramuscular; MSU: mid-stream urine

Remember to explain to patients that DMARDs take time to work – from one to six months, and that NSAIDs will be needed as well, especially at the beginning. Other treatments such as tumour necrosis factor (TNF) antagonists (etanercept and infliximab) reduce disease activity and joint inflammation more rapidly than DMARDs. Short-term toxicity is low, but long-term effects have yet to be observed.[9]

The expert patient and the health professional

RA is a chronic disease. The more patients know about the disease and how to manage it, the less overwhelmed they feel. Provide a contact address or website so that people can enquire at their own pace.[14] People with chronic debilitating illnesses need support and a secure relationship with at least one or two health professionals. Patient preference usually determines who those are. You should be able to explain:

- the importance of exercise in preventing loss of function
- physiotherapy as a possible treatment
- controlling weight to prevent excess load on joints
- how specialised footwear and podiatry can help
- drug treatment options
- the purpose of referral and what might be expected from the rheumatology or orthopaedic department.

The role of the GP or practice nurse also includes monitoring the general health of the patient. All involved in the care of the patient should consider the prevention and treatment of osteoporosis, the systemic effects of RA and the adverse effects of medication. Be alert for depression that can accompany any chronic illness, especially one that may cause social isolation through immobility. Other problems include loss of employment and low self-esteem. Physiotherapists and occupational therapists can help with advice on alternative ways of carrying out tasks, and aids to mobility or daily living. If there is much loss of function, employment modification or social service intervention may also be needed.

Case study 7.1 continued

Mr Stone is seen at the specialist assessment clinic for RA, has more blood tests and is started on methotrexate. He is referred back to you with the shared care protocol agreed with your PCO. With his consent, you write a report as requested by the occupational health doctor at his employing organisation, as they are trying to find ways of easing him back into work. You start making longer-term plans with him for modification of his lifestyle that had included a good deal of heavy manual work on the smallholding that he runs with his brother.

Osteoarthritis

Osteoarthritis is a heterogeneous condition that varies in the prevalence, risk factors, clinical features and prognosis, according to the joints affected. It most commonly affects knees, hips, spinal apophyseal joints and the hands. It is usually defined by the pathological or radiological appearance of the joints, rather than by the clinical features. Characteristically the cartilage surfaces of synovial joints show focal areas of damage together with remodelling of the underlying bone and mild synovitis. In severely affected joints, the joint space is narrowed and osteophytes form, with visible radiological subchondral bone changes.

   People usually start to have osteoarthritis between the ages of 45 and 55 years, and the prevalence increases with age. Only 5% of people below the age of 40 years will have any evidence of osteoarthritis, rising to 70% by the age of 75 years.[2] It is three times as common in women as men. The knee is the commonest site and affects 10% of the population aged over 50 years. Osteoarthritis of the hip is less common than of the knee, at less than 3% up to the age of 65 years, increasing to 5% of people aged over 80 years.

Case study 7.2

Mrs Wheeley complains to you that she has had to buy herself a shopping bag on wheels. 'Like an old lady, and I'm only 55', she grumbles. Her knees have become more and more painful recently and she is finding it difficult doing the shopping. The bus stop is at the bottom of the steep hill up to her house. She says that by the time she gets home her knees are so painful and swollen she has to have a rest before putting the shopping away. It has been coming and going for the last few years, but never as bad as now. She has some aches and pains elsewhere, and reminds you that she had a painful shoulder a few years ago that gradually improved, but is still not as good as it was. When you examine her knees, she jokes that they could win a knobbly-knees contest. They are both enlarged with a hard bony irregular feel and the right lower leg is at a slight angle to the upper leg, affecting her gait. Neither knee is red, but she is tender over the joint line. She cannot fully straighten or flex either knee.

What issues you should cover

Currently, diagnosis of OA is made on the structural changes detected either clinically or by the X-ray appearance. There is often discordance between the radiographic appearance and symptoms. The challenge for health professionals is to determine how much the radiographic changes (present so commonly in people especially over the age of 60 years) are contributing to the patient's overall problems. Box 7.1 gives a possible scheme for the assessment of the current clinical picture. Remember that you still need to think about other co-existing musculoskeletal disorders, even if someone has obvious osteoarthritis. Think about fibromyalgia, gout or pseudogout, RA, polymyalgia rheumatica and injury to ligaments or bursitis.

Box 7.1: Assessment of patients

Type of pain

- Mechanical: in OA, pain is worse with overuse.
- Inflammatory: stiffness and pain after rest in OA are usually short lived.
- Night pain: present but not severe in OA. If severe consider metastases or infection.

Ask about other symptoms

- Sleep disturbance: in OA it is usually the pain preventing the onset of sleep or causing waking with changes of position. Consider depression or fibromyalgia if early morning waking is prominent.
- Joint locking in OA may be present with a loose body, internal derangement or muscle weakness.
- Loss of function is more likely to be due to nerve or muscle conditions.
- There may be a history of a precipitating cause such as joint injury or disease.

Examination

- Is the pain in the joint (arthritis) or around it (peri-articular disease)?
- Are there painful points in the muscles as well (consider fibromyalgia)?

Management

The aims of treatment are:

- patient education
- control of pain
- improving function and quality of life
- avoidance of adverse effects of treatment
- minimising progression.

The Primary Care Rheumatology Society has drawn up guidelines on the management of osteoarthritis.[12]

NON-DRUG THERAPIES

Non-drug therapies for osteoarthritis include:[15]

- education about the condition and its management for patients, relatives and carers
- a positive attitude and information about the fact that most people with OA improve with time rather than deteriorate as they learn to manage better
- self-management programmes and contact with patient support organisations[14]
- social support by personal or telephone contact with other sufferers, volunteers, care-givers and professionals
- weight reduction if overweight
- exercise programmes
- walking aids
- modified footwear and other orthotic devices such as insoles or braces
- patellar taping
- modification of activities to protect joints
- aids to daily living
- acupuncture or electrotherapy.

For example, attending a day centre may enable someone to eat more wisely, lessen depression and isolation, and take exercise in an environment where many others are suffering in similar ways, improving quality of life and lessening pain and disability. Simple advice such as wearing supporting cushioned trainers on the feet may make an enormous difference to daily walking.

Case study 7.2 continued

You discuss with Mrs Wheeley how the pain and disability is affecting her life and what has made it worse recently. You discover that her son, who used to take her shopping in his car, has recently moved away with his young family. She becomes very tearful telling you how much she misses them. She reminds you that her husband died many years ago and her son was all she had. You suspect the move may have something to do with her over-involvement in her son's family. She has several symptoms suggestive of mild depression. You suggest that she might like a referral to the practice counsellor to try and make some positive plans to build up her own life, and she accepts with some doubts, but says that she doesn't want any pills for how she feels at present. You fix up an X-ray, make a plan for treatment and arrange to review her with the X-ray result.

Discuss diet and complementary therapies. Patients will try them out anyway, and you need to know what they are trying as part of the management plan. High vitamin C intake has been associated with a reduction in the progression of OA of the knee and lower vitamin D concentrations with faster progression of knee and hip OA, but there is no evidence yet of any benefit from vitamin supplements.[16] Chondroitin and glucosamine have been shown to be of some benefit at least in the short term, and the absence of side-effects makes them a popular choice for many patients.[16] Several studies have shown improvement in symptoms from the use of acupuncture.[2]

DRUG THERAPIES

Drug therapies for osteoarthritis should be used with caution, as many sufferers will have risk factors affecting the choice of medication. Conventional NSAIDs and Cox II inhibitors are probably overused. When they have been started because of severe pain and signs of inflammation, re-evaluate as soon as the pain and inflammation are under control, so that the patient can step down to simple analgesics as soon as possible. Systematic reviews have shown that simple analgesics and NSAIDs produce short-term relief of pain in osteo-arthritis, but there is no clear evidence of the superiority of NSAIDs (but listen to the individual patient; it is not your pain!). Consider safety, patient accept-ability and cost in your choice.[15] A pragmatic scheme is to step up or down depending on the level of pain:

- adequate doses of simple analgesics e.g. paracetamol
- topical preparations (NSAIDs, rubefacients, capsaicin)
- NSAIDs (only if symptoms are not controlled by other means or during acute flare-up; step down after control has been obtained)
- intra-articular corticosteroid injection (for acute flare-up or if the patient is unfit for surgery)
- intra-articular hyaluronan injections (an expensive option now available for patients unfit for surgery).

INTRA-ARTICULAR INJECTION OF THE KNEE

Studies of intra-articular injection of glucocorticoids or hyaluronan compared to placebo have shown some limited effectiveness.[15] In some trials, both the placebo and the active ingredient groups showed substantial improvements from the baseline measurements. Simple aspiration of the knee joint may be just as effective – but the evidence is lacking.

JOINT REPLACEMENT SURGERY

Constant pain, particularly at rest or at night, is often the deciding factor for joint replacement. Knee replacement surgery is effective at relieving pain and improving function.[15]

Case study 7.2 continued

Mrs Wheeley tells you that she is feeling a lot better about her knees, but she is still having disturbed nights and difficulty with her walking. Her X-ray shows considerable OA in the right knee with less on the left. You discuss with her a referral to the orthopaedic surgeon for consideration of knee replacement. She tells you that her son has already offered to pay for a private consultation and you arrange an appointment. She has decided not to see the practice counsellor because of the long waiting list. She has thought about what you said about building up her own life and has already joined the local Women's Institute on the suggestion of her neighbour who can give her a lift to the meetings. Her neighbour has also suggested taking her along to aquarobics (an exercise class in the shallow end of the local pool at the school) but she is still thinking about that. You encourage her to attend, saying it will help to build up her muscle strength and improve her flexibility.

Collecting data to demonstrate your learning, competence, performance and standards of service delivery

Example cycle of evidence 7.1

- Focus: clinical care
- Other relevant foci: relationships with patients; working with colleagues

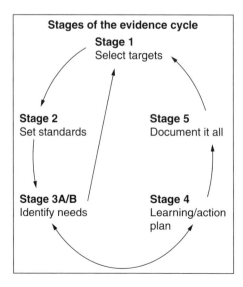

Stages of the evidence cycle

Stage 1
Select targets

Stage 2
Set standards

Stage 5
Document it all

Stage 3A/B
Identify needs

Stage 4
Learning/action plan

Case study 7.3

The practice secretary asks if you will speak to Ms Intense on the phone. She has rung frequently wanting many items of information and the practice secretary is finding her very difficult. You bring up the medical record and see Ms Intense has consulted your partner several times recently after moving into the area. She has been complaining of joint pains, fatigue, shortness of breath and difficulties with concentration. She has been off work for some time. A FBC, LFTs and biochemical screen were normal and ESR was only 2 mm/h. Your partner has put her down for further blood tests for SLE. Ms Intense tells you that she has already spoken to your partner about the tests required, but there is no entry in the record. She now wants to know if she will have a 'double-stranded DNA test'. She has contacted the Lupus Society,[17] and tells you that this is the best test to have. She sounds very anxious and convinced she has lupus despite your assurances that it is unlikely with the normal tests so far.

> This is just an example. Keep your task simple. You could choose three or four cycles of evidence to demonstrate your competence as a GP each year.

Stage 1: Select your aspirations for good practice

The excellent GP:

- keeps up to date
- works with colleagues to monitor the quality of the care provided
- communicates with colleagues and respects their skills and contributions
- records appropriate information for all contacts including telephone consultations
- gives patients the information they need about their problems in a way they can understand.

Stage 2: Set the standards for your outcomes

Outcomes might include:

- the way learning is applied
- a learnt skill
- a protocol
- a strategy that is implemented
- meeting recommended standards.

- Information about investigations is readily available to the practice team.
- Information about investigations can be communicated to patients in a way that they can understand.
- Co-operation between colleagues provides support for doctors.
- Telephone consultations are recorded in the medical record.

Stage 3A: Identify your learning needs

- Check whether you can find information about currently available investigations and when it was last updated.
- Compare your knowledge about SLE with that available on the lupus information site and other sources.[17,18]

Stage 3B: Identify your service needs

Any of the needs assessment exercises in 3A may also reveal service needs.

- Check whether the information about currently available investigations is available to other members of the practice team and whether it is in a form that is understandable to them.
- Find out what information is available to explain investigations to patients and whether it is up to date and can be understood by the majority.
- Ask at a practice meeting for a review of the health professionals' practice about recording telephone calls from and to patients and other contacts.
- Discuss with the practice secretary whether she is being asked to give information beyond her competence.
- Discuss with partners whether they feel able to ask for help with difficult consultations or situations.

Stage 4: Make and carry out a learning and action plan

- Plan an educational programme to suit your learning needs, learning style and what is available on types of arthritis and their investigation. Attend a lecture or course, a workshop, study day at the local postgraduate centre, or use an internet-based learning programme, read books, journals or internet-based research.
- Gather examples of good explanations of tests and investigations.
- Obtain up-to-date lists, or update those you have, of investigations available locally and more distantly, together with their indications and requirements.
- Ask the local educational tutor to arrange a talk by a local rheumatologist on what investigations are appropriate and useful in people with painful joints.
- At a practice team meeting arrange to discuss telephone encounters and when they should be recorded.
- Look at the way in which an adjacent practice, which you admire for its internal relations, organises mutual support for the staff and doctors. Arrange for their practice manager to give a talk to your practice team about how they do it.

Stage 5: Document your learning, competence, performance and standards of service delivery

- Document the educational events you have participated in and how they will affect the way in which you practise.
- Include a copy of the good explanations of tests and investigations and how they will be available to the practice team.
- Include the up-to-date list of investigations available locally and more distantly, together with their indications and requirements.
- Record how telephone encounters will be recorded in patient records.
- Include a summary of your visit to a nearby practice with an excellent reputation for the staff relationships, and the practice manager's visit to your practice, together with a record of key changes to the organisation of your own practice.

Case study 7.3 continued

You discuss the management of Ms Intense's anxiety about her health with your partner and how harm from excessive investigation can be avoided. You help to make a plan how to manage Ms Intense's demands on practice time and resources.

The practice team benefits from the greater knowledge about arthritis. They feel able to ask you for help in advising them on appropriate investigations and management.

Telephone calls are recorded more consistently in the patient records, improving team communication.

The practice team agrees that they will take it in turn to present a difficult management problem once a month after the business practice meeting, and at other times if there is an urgent need for support and co-operation between the team members to prevent harm. One of the practice nurses attends a facilitators' course, so that she can help to run the session more professionally.

Example cycle of evidence 7.2

- Focus: making effective use of resources
- Other relevant foci: good clinical care; relationships with patients; working with colleagues

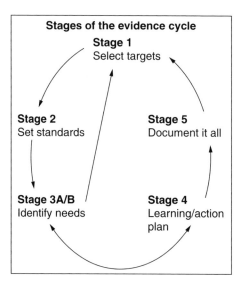

Stages of the evidence cycle

Stage 1
Select targets

Stage 2
Set standards

Stage 5
Document it all

Stage 3A/B
Identify needs

Stage 4
Learning/action plan

Case study 7.4

The receptionist gives you a request to renew the repeat prescription for Mr Lame. You are unfamiliar with the patient and look up his medical record. He has a repeat list including co-codamol, diclofenac, lansoprazole, folic acid and methotrexate. You cannot find a recent hospital letter, nor are there any recent blood results in his general practice record. You telephone him to find out what is happening about monitoring his treatment. He tells you that he has not been for his last three appointments at the hospital because they have sent car transport – and he cannot get in or out of an ordinary car. He has told them he needs transport with a lift, but this has been ignored. He cannot access the surgery either because he has a powered wheelchair that is too wide for the turn involved in accessing the treatment room. He was told that no one was available to take his blood at home. He has not had a blood test for eight months, although he is supposed to have them monthly. He sounds fed up.

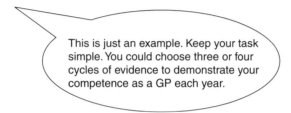

This is just an example. Keep your task simple. You could choose three or four cycles of evidence to demonstrate your competence as a GP each year.

Stage 1: Select your aspirations for good practice

The excellent GP:

- ensures that the repeat prescription system works safely
- audits the access for patients to the surgery premises
- ensures that health workers understand the needs of patients with disabilities for specialised transport
- provides sufficient health professionals able to carry out routine monitoring of medication
- has a system for following up patients who do not attend booked hospital appointments.

Stage 2: Set the standards for your outcomes

Outcomes might include:

- the way learning is applied
- a learnt skill
- a protocol
- a strategy that is implemented
- meeting recommended standards.

- The system for repeat prescriptions works safely.
- The practice premises are accessible to people with disabilities as far as possible, or the service is provided at patients' homes.

- Health workers are enabled to arrange appropriate transport for patients.
- Sufficient trained staff are available to provide services.
- A system for the follow-up of patients who fail to attend hospital appointments is in operation.

Stage 3A: Identify your learning needs

- Identify whether you know what monitoring patients on DMARDs require.
- Audit your own repeat prescription monitoring to discover how often you override the review date for patients whom you think you know.

Stage 3B: Identify your service needs

> Any of the needs assessment exercises in 3A may also reveal service needs.

- Audit the records of patients to establish how many patients on DMARDs are not being monitored correctly or safely.
- Ask Mr Lame if he will come to the surgery and take the practice manager around using his wheelchair to identify access problems. Repeat the process with other patients with other disabilities such as hearing, vision or intellectual capacity.
- Ask the practice manager to identify what training the health workers have had in arranging transport for patients, and find out how hospital staff make transport arrangements.
- Find out why Mr Lame was told there was no one available to take blood at home and how the situation can be changed.
- Find out whether the hospital always notifies the practice when patients do not attend, and what action is taken when notification is received.

Stage 4: Make and carry out a learning and action plan

- Update your knowledge of testing for DMARDS by going through the locally agreed guidelines for shared care.
- Reveal the results of your audit of repeat prescribing at a practice meeting, and discuss whether any changes need to be made generally.
- Work with the practice manager to establish accessible and appropriate transport for patients.
- Work with the practice manager to maximise access to services on practice premises.
- Work with the practice manager to train more staff in phlebotomy.

- Find out from other practices what they do when they are notified that patients have not attended hospital appointments; discuss this with the team and introduce new practice.

Stage 5: Document your learning, competence, performance and standards of service delivery

- You record that you have added the guidelines for monitoring DMARDs to a desktop file, and include a copy in your portfolio.
- Record the results of your audit of repeat prescribing at a practice meeting, and any changes made.
- Record what has been done to establish accessible and appropriate transport for patients.
- Record what has been done to maximise access to services on practice premises.
- Record how you have trained more staff in phlebotomy.
- Write down the system the practice has introduced to contact patients who have not attended hospital appointments.

Case study 7.4 continued

You discuss Mr Lame with your partner who usually looks after his care. She says that Mr Lame had always been so meticulous over his management she had assumed he was still managing everything himself, and was unaware of any problems. She contacted Mr Lame to offer her apologies and ask what could be done to improve his access problems.

You and the practice manager discover a good deal of ignorance about special needs transport and are able to institute a training plan for practice staff and propose one for the PCO. Representations are also made to the ambulance service to improve their liaison with the hospital staff responsible for booking transport.

Several of the nursing auxiliaries for the district nurse service are trained in phlebotomy to increase the availability of phlebotomy for people who cannot travel to the practice premises.

You and the practice manager find that it is possible to make some small changes in the layout of the practice premises to improve access, but Mr Lame still cannot manoeuvre his large chair round the sharp corners to the treatment room. He is pleased that he can now have his blood tests and see the practice nurse in one of the consulting rooms if it is arranged in advance.

The practice introduces a system of contacting patients to ask why they have not been able to attend hospital.

Example cycle of evidence 7.3

- Focus: clinical care
- Other relevant foci: relationships with patients; teaching and training; working with colleagues

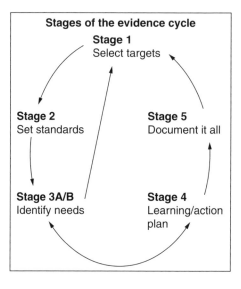

Stages of the evidence cycle

Stage 1
Select targets

Stage 2
Set standards

Stage 5
Document it all

Stage 3A/B
Identify needs

Stage 4
Learning/action plan

Case study 7.5

You have a medical student with you when Mrs Bellow is consulting about her weight and blood pressure. Just as she is leaving, she says 'Oh, and I needs a note to take for the housing so as we can have a bungalow'. You enquire some more and find that Mr Bellow cannot manage the stairs because of his arthritis and Mrs Bellow has been to the housing department at the Council Offices to ask to be moved from their council house. You arrange to visit Mr Bellow with the medical student. You find an equally overweight man of 68 years, who walks with difficulty with two wooden crook-handled sticks that he tells you belonged to his father. He spends most of his time sitting in a sagging armchair and uses a bucket hidden by the side of the chair for his urine output. Arrayed on a nearby table are a large assortment of food supplements and complementary medicines. You take the opportunity to show these to the medical student and point out that many people with arthritis spend a lot of money on these preparations. The medical student makes a list of them so that she can look up which ones have evidence of effectiveness.[9] You tell Mr and Mrs Bellow that you feel Mr Bellow needs an assessment by the occupational therapist so that he can be helped to be more independent and do more – and Mrs Bellow laughs heartily saying 'He never did nothing before. Can't see him doing much now his joints do hurt. He just shouts when he wants some't'.

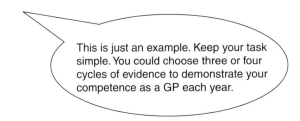

This is just an example. Keep your task simple. You could choose three or four cycles of evidence to demonstrate your competence as a GP each year.

Stage 1: Select your aspirations for good practice

The excellent GP:

- has a structured approach for managing long-term health problems
- only provides that which will make an effective contribution to the patient's overall management
- uses every opportunity to identify and use illustrations for teaching and training
- communicates effectively with others involved in the care of the patient.

Stage 2: Set the standards for your outcomes

Outcomes might include:

- the way learning is applied
- a learnt skill
- a protocol
- a strategy that is implemented
- meeting recommended standards.

- You can provide the evidence for the effectiveness or otherwise of complementary therapies.
- You have a contact list of professionals allied to medicine, what services they can provide and what information they require about patients.
- You have the skills to identify and communicate teaching points to others.

Stage 3A: Identify your learning needs

- Check that you and your practice are providing the necessary healthcare for people with arthritis.[12]
- Ask professionals allied to medicine to give you feedback about how well you communicate about patients.

- Ask for anonymised feedback on your teaching from the medical students you are allocated.

Stage 3B: Identify your service needs

> Any of the needs assessment exercises in 3A may also reveal service needs.

- Carry out a significant event review of Mr Bellow with the practice team to discover whether any deficiencies in care have resulted in his immobility.
- Undertake a SWOT analysis (*see* page 24) of services for people with arthritis in the practice.

Stage 4: Make and carry out a learning and action plan

- Ask the occupational therapist and the domiciliary physiotherapist to talk to the practice team about their services.
- Discuss the significant event audit of Mr Bellow and what changes need to be made.
- Identify what learning needs exist in the practice for managing the long-term care of people with arthritis, and start planning a learning programme.
- Attend a refresher course on teaching and training.

Stage 5: Document your learning, competence, performance and standards of service delivery

- Keep notes of the presentation by the occupational therapist and the domiciliary physiotherapist to the practice team about their services.
- Record the results of the significant event audit of Mr Bellow and what changes were agreed.
- Record what learning needs exist in the practice for managing the long-term care of people with arthritis, and the learning programme planned.
- Record your reflections about the refresher course on teaching and training.

Case study 7.5 continued

Mr Bellow is assessed by the occupational therapist and social services for the help he needs. He is resistant to any suggestion that he should make more effort to move, and the occupational therapist leaves a message saying he was 'quite blunt' about not requiring her help.

You are disappointed to hear that the medical student doesn't think general practice is what she wants to do, as she is more interested in technical medicine rather than 'all this social stuff'. However, your refresher course helps you to be realistic about passing on your own enthusiasm.

The practice team improves the general care of people with arthritis and you feel that patient needs are less likely to be missed in future.

References

1   Symmonds DP, Barrett EM, Bankhead CR *et al.* (1994) The incidence of rheumatoid arthritis in the United Kingdom: results from the Norfolk Arthritis Register. *British Journal of Rheumatology.* **33**: 735–9.

2   Snaith ML (ed.) (1999) *ABC of Rheumatology.* BMJ Books, London.

3   Yelin E, Henke C and Epstein W (1987) The work dynamic of the person with rheumatoid arthritis. *Arthritis and Rheumatism.* **30**: 507–12.

4   Mutru O, Laakso M, Isomki H and Koota K (1985) Ten year mortality and causes of death in patients with rheumatoid arthritis. *British Medical Journal.* **290**: 1811–13.

5   Members of the Ad Hoc Committee on Clinical Guidelines (1996) Guidelines for the initial evaluation of the adult patient with acute musculoskeletal symptoms. *Arthritis and Rheumatism.* **39**: 1–8.

6   Multi-disciplinary development group (2000) *Learning Guide for General Practitioners and General Practitioner Registrars.* Arthritis and Rheumatism Campaign, Chesterfield.

7   Arthritis Research Campaign (2003) *British National Formulary.* British Medical Association and Royal Pharmaceutical Society of Great Britain, London. www.bnf.org

8   NSAID Focus (1998) *Bandolier.* **52-2**. www.jr2.ox.ac.uk/bandolier/band52/b52-2.html

9   Godlee F (exec. ed.) (2003) *Clinical Evidence Concise.* **10**: 274–6. BMJ Publishing Group, London. www.clinicalevidence.com

10 Coxibs in Arthritis (2002 update) *Bandolier* www.jr2.ox.ac.uk/bandolier/booth/Arthritis/coxib702.html

11 McGhee M (2003) *A Guide to Laboratory Investigations* (4e). Radcliffe Medical Press, Oxford.

12 Foord-Kelcey G (ed.) (2004) *Guidelines.* **22**: 324–8. www.eguidelines.co.uk

13 Wakley G, Chambers R and Dieppe P (2001) *Musculoskeletal Matters in Primary Care.* Radcliffe Medical Press, Oxford.

14   Arthritis Research Campaign, St Mary's Court, St Mary's Gate, Chesterfield, Derbyshire S41 7TD; Tel: +44 (0)1246 558033. www.arc.org.uk

15   Godlee F (exec. ed.) (2003) *Clinical Evidence Concise.* **10:** 267–9. www.clinical evidence.com

16   Madhok R, Kerr H and Capell HA (2000) Recent advances: rheumatology. *British Medical Journal.* **321:** 882–5.

17   www.uklupus.co.uk

18   www.niams.nih.gov/hi/topics/lupus/slehandout

8

Osteoporosis

The main consequence of osteoporosis is the increased tendency to fracture with minor trauma and the subsequent loss of function and quality of life. Colles' fracture affects 15% of women and vertebral fractures up to 20% (although many are asymptomatic). Hip fracture affects one in four of women who live to 85 years, a quarter of whom die within 12 months and more than half remain disabled.[1]

Case study 8.1

You are surprised to see Mrs Gaunt, a 52-year-old woman, as she rarely consults for herself. Her husband has been on long-term sickness benefit and she works long hours as a caretaker at a local school. She tells you stiffly that her mother has just died aged 68 years, following a fall in the house when she broke her hip. The specialist at the hospital told her that her mother's bones had crumbled away and that she and her younger sister should have a bone scan.

What issues you should cover

Although the family history is one indicator of risk, you will want to find out how many risk factors Mrs Gaunt might have. For example:

- being female: females have an increased risk
- being elderly: she is not that yet
- early menopause: ask about when her periods stopped
- smoking: ask about previous and current use
- high alcohol intake: mainly because of decreased nutrition
- physical inactivity: this is unlikely given her employment
- thin body type: this you can observe

- heredity: establish if her mother had any particular risk factors that might not be inherited, such as one of the secondary causes in Box 8.1
- secondary osteoporosis (*see* Box 8.1).

Box 8.1:   Types of osteoporosis

Primary

- Type 1 (postmenopausal)
- Type 2 (age-related bone loss)
- Idiopathic (at ages less than 50 years)

Secondary

- Endocrine e.g. thyrotoxicosis, primary hyperparathyroidism, Cushing's syndrome
- Hypogonadism, from anorexia nervosa or excessive exercise
- Gastrointestinal e.g. malabsorption such as coeliac disease, partial gastrectomy, liver disease
- Rheumatological e.g. rheumatoid arthritis, ankylosing spondylitis
- Malignancy e.g. multiple myeloma, metastases
- Drugs e.g. corticosteroids, heparin

Bone scan investigations

Currently there is no rationale for population screening for low bone density. It makes sense to target those most likely to be at risk from the above lists. You might investigate a perimenopausal woman who has risk factors, to help her make a decision about using hormone replacement therapy. Similarly, you might wish to screen younger women with risk factors such as premature menopause or anorexia nervosa. Other indications would be those patients with diseases causing secondary osteoporosis (*see* Box 8.1), patients on more than 7.5 mg prednisolone or equivalent for more than 6 months, or those with a low impact fracture. Your local bone density screening unit is likely to have a list of criteria that Mrs Gaunt must satisfy before she can be screened, and it would be helpful to go through these with her to determine how much at risk she is.

Results of bone density scans

If osteoporosis (T score −1 to −2.5) or osteopenia (T score below −2.5) is found, you should screen for underlying causes with other investigations:

- serum calcium, phosphate, alkaline phosphatase, and creatinine
- serum protein electrophoresis
- thyroid function tests
- serum testosterone in men
- urinary Bence–Jones protein, or 24 hour urinary calcium or creatinine excretion as indicated by the clinical findings and consultation with the laboratory.

Treatment for those patients with osteopenia or osteoporosis

You would want to ensure that all patients at risk receive lifestyle advice, i.e. regular weight-bearing exercise, adequate nutrition including calcium and vitamin D, and avoidance of smoking or excess alcohol. Preventing falls minimises fracture risk and a useful summary of strategies appears in the *Drug and Therapeutics Bulletin* on managing falls in older people.[2] You will want to minimise other risk factors, but this may not be possible, e.g. for a patient needing steroid treatment. Education about osteoporosis for patients, carers and relatives is very helpful and the National Osteoporosis Society produces relevant material as well as providing a patient helpline.[3]

Pain relief for established osteoporosis is mainly by analgesic medication working up from paracetamol in full dosage to opiates. Remember that opiates or opiate-like drugs may increase the risk of falling. Low-dose antidepressants are useful for their pain-modulating effects and you might wish to refer to the pain clinic. Lumbar supports, transcutaneous nerve stimulators, or acupuncture are useful.

Drug treatments for improving bone mass (or preventing further loss) are summarised in the guidelines from the Royal College of Physicians,[4] and you could consider the medications in Table 8.1 for established osteoporosis or for osteopenia with a history of previous fracture.

Table 8.1:   Drugs to improve bone mass[4,5]

Drug	Guidelines
Vitamin D and calcium	Recommended daily dose 800 IU of vitamin D and 0.5–1 g of calcium. Has been shown to reduce hip fracture in frail elderly, modest reduction in non-vertebral fracture in men and women over 65 years. Usually used as adjuncts to other treatments
Calcium	At 1000 mg daily has a less marked effect than when given with vitamin D
Calcitriol, ergocalciferol, alphacalcidol	These vitamin D supplements given at pharmacological dosage require plasma calcium monitoring
Biphosphonates e.g. aledronate, etidronate, risenronate	Poor absorption means they should be taken on an empty stomach, but they can cause gastrointestinal problems. Once weekly dosage now available
Hormone replacement therapy e.g. oestrogen, testosterone	Treatment should be for at least five years to decrease the fracture risk, long-term treatment risks (e.g. increased cancer of breast or prostate) must be balanced against gains
Selective oestrogen receptor modulators (SERMS) e.g. raloxifene	SERMs like raloxifene are useful for those women who do not require relief of hot flushes, or who need to avoid the oestrogen-stimulating effect on the endometrium or breast
Calcitonin or teriparatide	Available as subcutaneous injection; it also has analgesic effects useful in acute fracture
Anabolic steroids	Androgenic side-effects make these unsuitable for women

Collecting data to demonstrate your learning, competence, performance and standards of service delivery

Example cycle of evidence 8.1

- Focus: complaints
- Other relevant foci: working with colleagues; teaching and training; relationships with patients

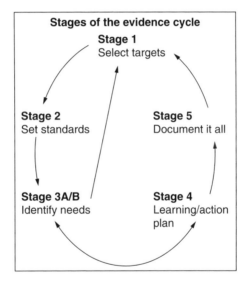

Stages of the evidence cycle

Stage 1
Select targets

Stage 2
Set standards

Stage 5
Document it all

Stage 3A/B
Identify needs

Stage 4
Learning/action plan

Case study 8.2

Your practice has received a patient complaint about the GP retainer. Mrs Faddy, who has coeliac disease, had fallen and sustained a Colles' fracture. A doctor at the hospital had commented that she should have been put on bone protective medication. Looking through the medical records, Mrs Faddy had attended the GP retainer on several occasions complaining about how difficult it was to stick to the diet, but there did not appear to have been any discussion of the osteoporosis risk.

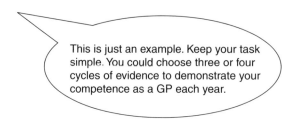

This is just an example. Keep your task simple. You could choose three or four cycles of evidence to demonstrate your competence as a GP each year.

Stage 1: Select your aspirations for good practice

The excellent GP:

- apologises appropriately when things go wrong, and has an adequate complaints procedure in place
- makes sure that colleagues in training posts receive appropriate supervision.

Stage 2: Set the standards for your outcomes

> Outcomes might include:
>
> - the way learning is applied
> - a learnt skill
> - a protocol
> - a strategy that is implemented
> - meeting recommended standards.

- Understand and establish effective processes for preventing and managing complaints from patients in the practice.
- Ensure that health professionals in training posts have adequate supervision and opportunities for keeping up to date.

Stage 3A: Identify your learning needs

- Examine as a significant event one or more complaints, e.g. where the practice has not advised a patient correctly about the complaints process.
- Compare the actual care of a patient against an acceptable standard of care for patients with coeliac disease. Use peer review by asking respected colleagues or compare your practice against a published standard such as a guideline by a responsible body of professional opinion.[6]

Stage 3B: Identify your service needs

Any of the needs assessment exercises in 3A may also reveal service needs.

- Audit patient complaints in the preceding 12 months: the number, the outcomes and how the complaint system is advertised, etc.
- Audit the extent to which doctors and nurses are following practice agreed protocols. This is about being proactive about preventing or minimising the likelihood of the source of the complaint recurring.
- Audit vulnerable areas. Look back at the analysis of complaints to identify useful areas for focusing learning, e.g. a review the use of bone protective agents in people prescribed oral steroids.
- Review the way that the GP retainer is offered supervision and how her personal and professional development plan is being implemented.

Stage 4: Make and carry out a learning and action plan

- Ask your PCO to look at the practice complaints system and feed back on how it can be improved (if at all).
- Arrange a tutorial between the practice manager and others in the team about preventing and managing complaints, or use one of the risk management packages produced by medical defence organisations.[7,8]
- Read up on how to undertake significant event analysis including how to share the information with the practice team and respond as a practice team.
- Find out how to add a reminder to the records of patients at risk of osteoporosis.

Stage 5: Document your learning, competence, performance and standards of service delivery

- Keep a copy of how the complaint was managed.
- Produce a protocol of the patient complaint process against which consecutive complaints can be audited in another 12 months' time.
- Keep a record of how the GP retainer will be supervised and how she will be helped with her personal and professional development plan.
- Record how you added a reminder to the records of patients with risk factors for osteoporosis.

Case study 8.2 continued

Mr and Mrs Faddy meet with the practice manager, the GP retainer and yourself. During the discussion, it becomes apparent that Mrs Faddy blames herself for failing to stick to the diet, while Mr Faddy is angry that he had not been aware of the importance of the condition, believing it no more than a fussy diet. Since the complaint, a bone scan arranged by the hospital has not shown any osteoporosis and Mr and Mrs Faddy are cross with the hospital doctor for alarming them so much. The GP retainer says she will learn more about coeliac disease and spend some time passing on her knowledge to the couple. You rearrange regular meetings with the GP retainer that had been allowed to lapse due to pressure of work.

Example cycle of evidence 8.2

- Focus: keeping good records
- Other relevant foci: maintaining good medical practice; prescribing; working with colleagues

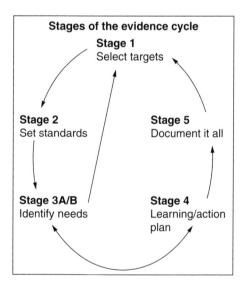

Stages of the evidence cycle

Stage 1
Select targets

Stage 2
Set standards

Stage 5
Document it all

Stage 3A/B
Identify needs

Stage 4
Learning/action plan

Case study 8.3

Mrs Dirge is not a welcome name on your patient list. She consults frequently but has so many things wrong with her that it is difficult to know how to manage any one complaint. She has hypertension, diabetes, chronic obstructive pulmonary disease, osteoarthritis and has recently developed polymyalgia rheumatica, and was prescribed high-dose steroids. She usually consults your partner who has been on sick leave for two months and you feel a momentary irritation that here is another burden for those left to cope. Among several other complaints, she wants something for indigestion and says she could not take the tablets one of your colleagues had recently given her. Looking at her recent prescription list, you see that she has had several different antacid medications repeated, two different proton pump inhibitors, is still taking naproxen as well as prednisolone and has stopped the Didronel PMO pack (disodium etidronate and calcium carbonate).

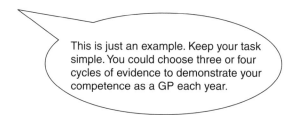

This is just an example. Keep your task simple. You could choose three or four cycles of evidence to demonstrate your competence as a GP each year.

Stage 1: Select your aspirations for good practice

The excellent GP:

- makes sound management decisions which are based on good practice and evidence
- records appropriate information for all contacts
- only prescribes treatments that make an effective contribution to the patient's overall management.

Stage 2: Set the standards for your outcomes

Outcomes might include:

- the way learning is applied
- a learnt skill
- a protocol
- a strategy that is implemented
- meeting recommended standards.

- The practice has an effective repeat prescribing policy that is consistently applied.
- The practice has an agreed policy for managing the needs of patients when the usual doctor responsible is absent.

Stage 3A: Identify your learning needs

- Note in your reflective diary your concerns about the repeat prescribing, the lack of overall control and the inappropriate use of antacids.
- Obtain feedback from 10 patients who usually see your absent partner about how their medical needs are being managed, to determine whether your irritation and overwork (and that of your partners) is affecting their care.

Stage 3B: Identify your service needs

> Any of the needs assessment exercises in 3A may also reveal service needs.

- Arrange for an anonymous comment form about repeat prescribing and how it works in practice to be completed by staff members involved.
- Conduct a SWOT analysis of repeat prescribing by the practice team, with a subsequent action plan to update or revise current practice policy.
- Arrange an audit of the adherence of the practice team to the repeat prescribing policy.
- Identify whether more health professional time is needed to manage patient need.

Stage 4: Make and carry out a learning and action plan

- Meet up with a pharmaceutical advisor to discuss repeat prescribing policy and the prescribing of antacids, gastroprotection for patients on steroids and NSAIDs and the best use of biphosphonates for bone protection. Meet the advisor on your own or with practice colleagues.
- Attend a workshop on the management of multiple medication.
- Discuss the audit and/or SWOT analysis results, proposed revisions to practice repeat prescribing in general, and the suggestions from the prescribing advisor to agree revisions to the practice protocol for repeat prescribing.

Stage 5: Document your learning, competence, performance and standards of service delivery

- Keep extracts from your reflective diary about the difficulties and the changes made to remedy them.
- Record the actions to increase health professional time available to manage patient need.

- Include the results of the audit, SWOT analysis and notes from the meeting with the prescribing advisor and the action plan that followed.
- Include a copy of the revised repeat prescribing policy.

Case study 8.3 continued

You explain briefly to Mrs Dirge that her medication is upsetting her stomach but that some of it is essential. You give her the repeat prescription slip with one of the proton pump inhibitors highlighted, and ask her to take that very regularly to protect her stomach. You ask her to fill a carrier bag with all the medication she has been given and bring it to another (longer) appointment with her to go through it all and rationalise it. You make a note to go through her records and make sure that she is not taking anything that she does not have to take in order to reduce the risk of iatrogenic symptoms.

Example cycle of evidence 8.3

- Focus: research
- Other relevant focus: clinical care

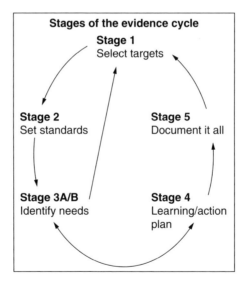

Stages of the evidence cycle

Stage 1
Select targets

Stage 2
Set standards

Stage 5
Document it all

Stage 3A/B
Identify needs

Stage 4
Learning/action plan

Case study 8.4

A new professor of rheumatology has taken up post at your local university. He has started several research projects. He is actively recruiting patients for his various trials and asks your practice to refer patients to his team. He needs patients with risk factors for osteoporosis for a trial of a new treatment. You can see that patients will benefit from the speedy referral process for bone density measurement.

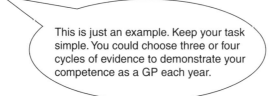

This is just an example. Keep your task simple. You could choose three or four cycles of evidence to demonstrate your competence as a GP each year.

Stage 1: Select your aspirations for good practice

The excellent GP:

- protects patients' rights and makes sure that they are not disadvantaged by taking part in research
- has information available on laws and requirements (e.g. research ethics) relating to general practice.

Stage 2: Set the standards for your outcomes

Outcomes might include:

- the way learning is applied
- a learnt skill
- a protocol
- a strategy that is implemented
- meeting recommended standards.

- The practice has a policy for GPs and staff undertaking research.
- You have library and patient literature on osteoporosis.

Stage 3A: Identify your learning needs

- Find out whether paper-based resources (e.g. books or files) or electronic sites describing best practice in management of osteoporosis are easily accessed by you in your practice.
- Reflect on whether you are up to date with current requirements for undertaking research or participating in someone else's research study. Decide

whether you are clear about research governance, what studies require ethics approval, how you obtain your trust's permission to host research, what information patients need before giving their consent to participate in research, etc.

Stage 3B: Identify your service needs

Any of the needs assessment exercises in 3A may also reveal service needs.

- Compare best practice in treating osteoporosis with the interventions that the university research team are comparing in their research. Seek an independent view (e.g. another specialist from outside the trial) as to whether patients will be disadvantaged by you referring them to the trial, remembering the benefits of a speedy referral process.
- Ask the PCO for a copy of the algorithm describing research governance management systems and guidance on how they affect you. Discuss with others in the practice what systems you need to develop to link into the new NHS requirements.
- Ask several patients to comment on the trial's patient information leaflet, to check that it is suitable for patients in your population.

Stage 4: Make and carry out a learning and action plan

- Meet up with research governance manager for a tutorial on research ethics and research governance systems. Compose a policy for practice staff to fit the legal and NHS requirements.
- Write out what constitutes best practice in investigating patients at risk of osteoporosis and the treatment of osteoporosis. Then compare previous treatment with the next case of each that presents and add notes about any subsequent change of treatment.
- Attend a seminar by the university research team introducing their research plans, and put specific questions and queries to the team.
- Compile a list of library or other resources (paper/electronic) your practice needs to buy so that there is sufficient reference material available in relation to osteoporosis and research ethics. Check your choice with a local health librarian if possible and place an order.

Stage 5: Document your learning, competence, performance and standards of service delivery

- Keep a copy of the practice policy on GPs and staff undertaking research.

- List the contents of the reference library in the practice and the resources available in each consulting room (e.g. paper and electronic versions of *Clinical Evidence*).[9]
- Keep a copy of the research ethics approval and details of the research study in which you intend to participate.
- Record the questions and answers from the research seminar.
- Keep the checklist of best practice in the investigation of patients at risk of osteoporosis and treatment of osteoporosis.

Case study 8.4 continued

After your preparations in understanding and preparing for participating in the research study, all goes smoothly. Patients are happy with the information leaflet about the trials and most consent to join in. Nearly all the local GPs and practices co-operate to refer suitable patients so that the research study is sufficiently powerful to be able to provide conclusive evidence of relative benefits of the treatments being compared.

References

1   Snaith ML (ed.) (1999) *ABC of Rheumatology*. BMJ Books, London.

2   Drugs and Therapeutics Bulletin (2000) Managing falls in older people. *Drugs and Therapeutics Bulletin.* **38**: 68–72.

3   National Osteoporosis Society, PO Box 10, Radstock, Bath BA3 3YB, UK. Patient helpline tel: +44 (0)1761 472721.

4   Royal College of Physicians, Bone and Tooth Society of Great Britain (2000) *Osteoporosis. Clinical guidelines for prevention and treatment. Update of pharmacological interventions and an algorithm for management*. Royal College of Physicians of London, London.

5   Compston J (2000) Updated guidelines on osteoporosis include management algorithm. *Guidelines in Practice.* **3**: 23–8.

6   British Society of Gastroenterology (2000) *Guidelines for Osteoporosis in Coeliac Disease and Inflammatory Bowel Disease*. British Society of Gastoenterology, London. www.eguidelines.co.uk

7   MPS Risk Consulting, Granary Wharf House, Leeds LS11 5PY, UK. www.mps-riskconsulting.com

8   MDU Services Ltd, 230 Blackfriars Road, London SE1 8PJ, UK. www.the-mdu.com

9   www.clinicalevidence.com

9

Back pain

Acute low back pain

> **Case study 9.1**
>
> Mr Wrench comes to see you in great pain. He was digging in the garden two days before and fine at the time except for a twinge of pain. He went inside, sat in his armchair and watched television. When he came to get up he found he was in agony and could not get out of his chair or get comfortable. In all his 40 years he has never known such pain. The emergency doctor was called who sympathised and left him a prescription for some co-codamol. The pain is slightly better and he is able to move but he cannot stand up straight and cannot bend down.
>
> You examine him and find that the pain is in the lumbo-sacral region, centrally sited without any radiation into the thighs. He has no numbness, tingling or weakness.

What issues you should cover

Acute low back pain is common and usually resolves spontaneously

You will want to tell Mr Wrench how common low back pain is. About three-quarters of people in developed countries will experience low back pain at some time in their lives.[1,2] Overall about 16.5 million people in the UK suffer from back pain in any one year. Most people can deal with their back pain themselves most of the time.[3] In a typical year, about three to seven million back pain sufferers are thought to consult a GP about their back pain at least once, 1.6 million people attend hospital-based outpatients, about 100 000 are admitted to hospital and 24 000 have surgery for back pain. About 7% of the adult population in the UK present to their GP with back pain in any one year.[3]

In most cases of acute low back pain, the pain resolves spontaneously within a few weeks, despite being severe at onset (acute low back pain is defined as lasting for less than six weeks). One research review found that four-fifths of people initially off work with acute low back pain had returned to work within a month.[4] Once a person has been off work with back pain for six months, they have about a 50% chance of getting back to work.[3] Three-quarters of people suffering acute low back pain have a recurrence within 12 months.

Simple acute low back pain is generally felt in the lumbo-sacral region as for Mr Wrench. It may be felt in the buttocks or thighs instead or as well as the lower back.

Look out for serious spinal conditions or nerve root compression

'Simple backache' describes back pain with a mechanical origin. That is, the pain originates from the bony structure of the spine or the muscles attached to it. Symptoms vary with different physical activities and time of day. Simple backache can be very painful; the pain may spread in a general way down to one or both hips, thighs and legs. The difference between simple backache and other types of back pain is that the lumbar or sciatic nerve roots or the spinal cord are not compressed. Box 9.1 describes the usual features of people with simple backache. Most cases of acute low back pain are due to mechanical factors, but for one in every 20 patients, the low back pain will arise from serious spinal pathology (1%) or nerve root compression (4%).[5]

Box 9.1:   Features of simple backache[6]
- Onset is usually between the ages of 20 and 55 years.
- Pain is in the lumbo-sacral region, buttocks and thighs.
- Pain is mechanical in nature: it varies with physical activity and over time.
- The individual is otherwise well.
- The outlook is good: 90% recover from an acute attack in six weeks.

Management in primary care

Patients with back pain should remain active, and bed rest should be discouraged.[1,3,5,6]

Take a history and examine the patient to rule out possible serious conditions or 'red flags' that would indicate possible serious spinal pathology (*see* Box 9.2). Mr Wrench does not seem to have any of these warning symptoms or signs.

Box 9.2:   Red flags[6,7]
- Presentation under age 20 years or onset over 55 years
- Non-mechanical pain
- Thoracic pain (possible dissecting aneurysm)
- Past history of steroids (possible osteoporotic vertebral collapse) or HIV
- Unwell, weight loss or history of carcinoma (possible metastases)
- Widespread neurological symptoms or signs
- Fever (possible osteomyelitis)
- Structural deformity
- Sphincter disturbance, gait disturbance or saddle anaesthesia indicating the cauda equina syndrome, which would warrant an emergency referral

---

Most patients with acute low back pain can be managed in primary care.[8] If you diagnose simple back pain, advise the patient about their posture, simple exercise, avoiding lifting heavy weights, and maintaining normal activities. Reinforce your advice with information leaflets. Suggest simple analgesics taken regularly, such as paracetamol or NSAIDs.

The evidence for encouraging physical therapies and exercise is good.[1,9] Continuing ordinary everyday activities leads to the most speedy recovery and least time off work; a planned return to normal work within a short time leads to less time off work in the long run. Manipulation provides short-term improvement in pain and activity for acute and subacute back pain; risks of complications are low. Exercise programmes can improve pain and functioning in people with chronic low back pain. There is no evidence that specific back exercises, such as aerobic or strengthening exercises, are more effective than other conservative treatments in acute low back pain. Ice, heat, and massage may all be used for relieving symptoms of pain and stiffness of the back, but do not appear to have any effect on speeding up recovery.

Acute back pain is usually due to conditions that cannot be diagnosed on a straight X-ray (except osteoporotic collapse). Routine X-rays are not recommended for investigating an acute episode of low back pain lasting less than six weeks, unless there are unusual signs that alert the doctor or therapist to the possibility of a serious disease. Three standard X-ray views of the lumbar spine involve 120 to 150 times the radiation dose of a chest X-ray and should not be undertaken lightly. An estimated 19 deaths may arise from the 700 000 people in the UK who have lumbar spine radiographs each year.[10] The GP cited in Box 9.3 explains that in his local guidelines it is never warranted for a GP to arrange a lumbar–sacral X-ray and that an MRI scan might be more appropriate, depending on the features.

Box 9.3: X-ray is not needed in most back pain: a GP gives sensible advice to other GPs about avoiding lumbar spine X-rays

'For the overwhelming majority of patients with back pain, X-ray is unnecessary and for those who warrant investigation, it is often not the imaging technique of choice. Lumbar spine X-rays generate a large quantity of radiation straight into the pelvis and EU regulations are very strict about the referrer's responsibility for ensuring that the benefits of exposure outweigh the risks. Certain groups of patients do need an X-ray, but for many, an MRI is the investigation of choice.

In my area, we no longer allow GPs to refer patients for lumbar spine X-rays. Patients with red flags should be referred urgently for an orthopaedic opinion, and the rest managed in primary care. For those who do not settle in the predicted fashion, we recommend referral to our extended-scope physiotherapy clinic, where a full assessment is carried out. If the clinical signs then warrant investigation, the physiotherapists refer for MRI. If this is normal, they can proceed with treatment. If not, a fast-track orthopaedic opinion is arranged without the need for further input.

This system works well as long as everybody plays their part. In particular, patients need to understand the place of self-care and education, and GPs need to be confident most patients do not need a further opinion, never mind an X-ray.'[11]

Referral to a specialist in secondary care

Mr Wrench appears to have simple backache, but if he had any signs of serious pathology he would need prompt investigation or referral in the next few weeks. The current guidelines from NICE are given in Box 9.4.[5] These summarise the symptoms, signs and timing for when patients with acute low back pain should be referred to a specialist.

Box 9.4: Referral advice for acute low back pain: summary of NICE guidance[5]

**** Neurological features of cauda equina syndrome (***immediately***, for sphincter disturbance, progressive motor weakness, perineal anaesthesia, or evidence of bilateral nerve root involvement)

*** Serious spinal pathology is suspected (***urgently***, preferably seen within 1 week)

*** The patient develops progressive neurological deficit (weakness, anaesthesia) (***urgently***, preferably seen within 1 week)

*** The patient has nerve root pain that is not resolving after 6 weeks (***urgently***, preferably seen within 3 weeks)

** An underlying inflammatory disorder such as ankylosing spondylitis is suspected (***soon***)

** The patient has simple back pain and has not resumed their normal activities in 3 months (***soon***). The effects of pain will vary and could

> include reduced quality of life, functional capacity, independence or
> psychological wellbeing. Where possible, referral should be to a multi-
> disciplinary back pain team.

Case study 9.1 continued

You reassure Mr Wrench that there is nothing to worry about. Backache is very
common. You tell him that there is no sign of any serious damage or disease. He
should expect a full recovery within weeks. Activity is helpful, too much rest is
not, and he should get back to his office work as soon as possible. As luck would
have it, the physiotherapist down the corridor is free, as another patient has not
turned up for their appointment. She gives Mr Wrench some further advice and
written information about exercise, and shows Mr Wrench how to do the
extension exercises she recommends.

Chronic non-specific low back pain

Case study 9.2

Mr Crook has come to see you about his chronic low back pain – for the third
time in six months. He has been a warehouseman for 25 years, since he left
school. He has rarely had any time off work, but he is just very tired from
struggling to work despite his chronic low back pain making it difficult for him
to sleep or lift unwieldy packages. He breezes into the consulting room, walking
normally. When you examine him, he indicates that the pain radiates down his
left leg to his foot and straight leg raising of the left leg triggers the pain. He is
otherwise well.

What issues you should cover

Back pain and arthritis are the two most common reasons for chronic pain.[12]
About 6% of the population report low back pain lasting for at least a year.
Chronic back pain is variably defined as back pain that persists for longer than
7–12 weeks or 'pain that lasts beyond the expected period of healing'.[2,13] Data
about the epidemiology of chronic low back pain are uncertain. Five to ten per
cent of the population in the UK continue to have some degree of back pain
over long periods of their lives. Three to four per cent of the population aged 16

to 44 years, and 5–7% of those aged 45 to 64 years report back problems as a 'chronic sickness'.[14] Chronic back pain is sometimes used as a diagnosis of convenience by people who are actually disabled for socio-economic, work-related, or psychological reasons.[13]

Source of pain

Nerve root pain is usually caused by a disc prolapse, spinal stenosis or scarring from previous surgery which is causing compression of a nerve. Sciatica arises when the sciatic nerve root is compressed, as in Mr Crook's case. The pain from the compressed nerve root is localised to a particular site down one leg, which corresponds with the skin ending of that strand of the nerve. Sciatic pain commonly radiates down one leg to the foot or toes, following the path of the left or right branch of the sciatic nerve from the lumbar and sacral spine to the foot on the same side of the body. Numbness, and pins and needles are often associated with the distribution of the pain. Sometimes sensation is lost around the same area, or the muscle is weaker or the reflex of the muscle brisker.

Management

You will aim to lessen any disability and relieve Mr Crook's pain, without triggering side-effects from any drugs. You will encourage him to develop as positive an attitude as possible so that his chronic pain does not dominate his life unduly.

A great deal of research has been undertaken in relation to the effectiveness of drug and non-drug treatments or interventions. Look at *Clinical Evidence* for more information,[1] but these are summarised in Box 9.5.

Box 9.5: Likelihood that interventions for chronic low back pain and sciatica are beneficial[1]

Beneficial

- Exercise versus other treatments improves pain and functional status
- Intensive multidisciplinary biopsychosocial rehabilitation can reduce pain and improve function

Likely to be beneficial

- Analgesics such as paracetamol and tramadol can decrease pain and increase function
- Back school programmes can improve pain and reduce disability
- Behavioural therapy can reduce pain, improve function and behavioural outcomes
- Massage can reduce pain and improve a person's functioning

- NSAIDs such as naproxen increase pain relief
- Injections of trigger points or ligaments with a steroid plus local anaesthetic may relieve pain, as may a phenol injection of the lumbar interspinal ligament

Unknown or conflicting effectiveness

- Acupuncture at traditional acupuncture points or at trigger sites for the pain; needles may be stimulated manually or electrically
- Antidepressant drugs: beneficial effects on pain relief, but not necessarily depression or function
- Electromyographic biofeedback
- Epidural steroid injection
- Lumbar support such as lumbar corset
- Muscle relaxant
- Spinal manipulation
- Transcutaneous electrical nerve stimulation

Likely to be ineffective or harmful

- Facet joint injection such as with an intra-articular corticosteroid injection – potential harm may arise from pain, infection, haemorrhage or neurological damage or chemical meningitis
- Traction – potential harm may arise from loss of muscle tone, thrombophlebitis, bone demineralisation and debilitation.

Be positive about managing pain. New national guidelines in Australia have issued advice about avoiding 'alarming' or 'inappropriate' terms such as 'degeneration' and 'rupture' and substituting 'wear and tear' and 'prolapsed' instead, in the case of acute back pain and musculoskeletal pain.[15] The project leader is reported to have said 'I feel it's an awful thing for a doctor to tell a patient they have a "ruptured" disc. They imagine they have their disc splattered on the inside of their spinal cord ... If you don't explain to patients relatively quickly and have a pretty good idea what the diagnosis is ... then they are the patients who will slip over to become chronic pain patients'.

Some psychological factors are associated with an increased risk of chronic low back pain. Negative attitudes and beliefs and behaviours on the part of the person with back pain may predict poor outcomes.[16]

Case study 9.2 continued

Mr Crook decides to take your advice to try regular exercise again – it had helped in the past, but his enthusiasm has lapsed and he has felt too tired to go out again to exercise after work. He starts swimming and cycling (with the saddle raised) regularly, and is amazed by the beneficial effects this has on reducing his back pain and sciatica and his mood in general. He is very careful how he lifts at work, bending his knees, keeping objects close to his body with his back straight, then lifting by straightening his knees rather than his back. Next time he comes to see you in surgery it is for something other than his back pain.

Collecting data to demonstrate your learning, competence, performance and standards of service delivery

Example cycle of evidence 9.1

- Focus: practice management/good employer practices
- Other relevant foci: manual handling; learning culture

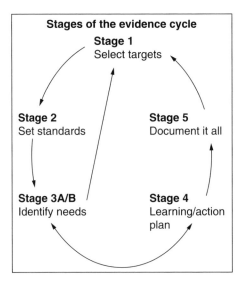

Stages of the evidence cycle

Stage 1 Select targets

Stage 2 Set standards

Stage 5 Document it all

Stage 3A/B Identify needs

Stage 4 Learning/action plan

Case study 9.3

As the education lead for your practice team, you are concerned about whether everyone knows how and whether they should be lifting weights, after one of the receptionists goes off sick having pulled her back at work, carrying boxes of photocopier paper.

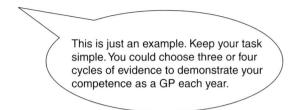

This is just an example. Keep your task simple. You could choose three or four cycles of evidence to demonstrate your competence as a GP each year.

Stage 1: Select your aspirations for good practice

The excellent GP:

- learns from mistakes
- is a good employer in respect of manual handling at work.

Stage 2: Set the standards for your outcomes

Outcomes might include:

- the way learning is applied
- a learnt skill
- a protocol
- a strategy that is implemented
- meeting recommended standards.

- You and other practice colleagues adhere to manual handling policy.
- Establish a culture in your practice where staff learn from mistakes.

Stage 3A: Identify your learning needs

- Assess any lifting you, or staff who work with you, are involved in at work against the legal requirements of current manual handling regulations. Weigh loads that you or they might typically lift and see how they match weight limits in the regulations.
- Ask the community physiotherapist to watch you lift a load or package and comment on your technique. Repeat with other staff with whom you work.
- Keep a reflective diary for a month and note down any mistakes, and ways in which the possibility of recurrences might be avoided or minimised. Check at the end of the reflective period whether action was taken to minimise recurrences or share learning from mistakes with others.

Stage 3B: Identify your service needs

> Any of the needs assessment exercises in 3A may also reveal service needs.

- Find out whether your practice has a manual handling policy. If not, derive one from other sources (another practice, your PCO). If so, check that the contents of the manual handling policy conform to best practice.[9]
- Undertake a risk assessment of hazards or lifting that cannot be avoided in the practice, in everyday work or when stationery or water carriers are delivered, etc.
- Review the staff injury arrangements – are all such injuries logged, is the incident handled properly, is subsequent action taken to prevent recurrence?

Stage 4: Make and carry out a learning and action plan

- Read up on good practice in manual handling.[9] Write and agree, or update the practice policy on manual handling.
- Attend an updating session from the physiotherapist assistant on manual handling, or watch a training video and practise lifting correctly afterwards.
- Talk to colleagues in neighbouring practices over coffee at a workshop on an unrelated topic, about ways they learn from mistakes or critical incidents. Discuss with the practice team setting up a regular learning session involving review of significant events or critical incidents occurring in the practice.

Stage 5: Document your learning, competence, performance and standards of service delivery

- Include a copy of the practice manual handling policy.
- Keep notes from the monthly review of significant events and critical incidents, and the action taken to minimise recurrence.
- Arrange and record an audit of the way manual handling policy is applied through observation of everyday practice by the physiotherapist, three months later.

Case study 9.3 continued

The receptionist is back at work after a few days, though still grumbling about her back. The physiotherapist organises for a colleague to come into the practice one lunchtime to give everyone a refresher on how they should lift boxes or other awkward packages, and sensible weight limits.

Example cycle of evidence 9.2

- Focus: complementary medicine
- Other relevant foci: clinical care; evidence-based practice

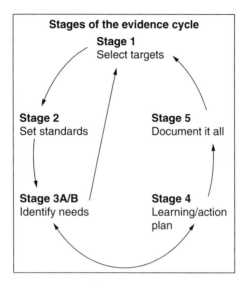

Case study 9.4

Ms Hope consults you to ask for advice about what complementary medicine techniques she might try to help her back pain, as the conventional drugs you have tried (paracetamol and ibuprofen) do not give her enough pain relief. She wants to know if acupuncture, glucosamine or massage are safe and worth trying.

This is just an example. Keep your task simple. You could choose three or four cycles of evidence to demonstrate your competence as a GP each year.

Stage 1: Select your aspirations for good practice

The excellent GP:

- knows about the nature and reliability of common treatments, whether they are conventional or complementary treatments
- maintains his or her knowledge and skills, and is aware of his or her limits of competence.

Stage 2: Set the standards for your outcomes

Outcomes might include:

- the way learning is applied
- a learnt skill
- a protocol
- a strategy that is implemented
- meeting recommended standards.

- Be able to explain the evidence base for interventions that give benefits for low back pain.

Stage 3A: Identify your learning needs

- Self-assess your knowledge of the benefits/risks of complementary treatments, especially acupuncture and glucosamine, and massage for back pain.
- Try to find reliable evidence about the complementary interventions in question within five minutes – either from the PC in your consulting room or a nearby book. Do you know the websites or publication to access easily for the evidence base?[17]
- Once you have learnt enough about the effectiveness of these interventions (*see* Stage 4) explain the evidence to the patient – and then ask for feedback from the patient as to whether they understood your explanation or have any more questions.

Stage 3B: Identify your service needs

Any of the needs assessment exercises in 3A may also reveal service needs.

- Check whether there is any patient literature about self-care of back pain in the waiting room or consulting rooms. Does it cover complementary treatments? Do you or others in the team know any websites covering self-care, to which patients can be directed ?[18]
- Find out what local services exist to provide acupuncture or massage through the NHS or privately.

Stage 4: Make and carry out a learning and action plan

- Read up about the effectiveness of interventions for acute and chronic back pain from a reliable source.[1,7,17]
- Read patient literature that you have accessed from reliable websites.[18]

Stage 5: Document your learning, competence, performance and standards of service delivery

- Photocopy the evidence for treatments for back pain in your portfolio or folder so that it can be easily consulted in future if other patients ask you the same questions about the effectiveness of complementary treatments.
- Include copies of the relevant patient literature.

Case study 9.4 continued

Ms Hope listens to the evidence you relay that the effectiveness of acupuncture and massage is unknown as regards back pain, and similarly, that there is some evidence that glucosamine may be beneficial for osteoarthritis, but the evidence is not yet conclusive. She decides to give acupuncture a go, as it seems reasonably safe to do so, and finds that her pain subsides considerably as a result.

Example cycle of evidence 9.3

- Focus: relationships with patients
- Other relevant foci: clinical care; teamwork; evidence-based practice

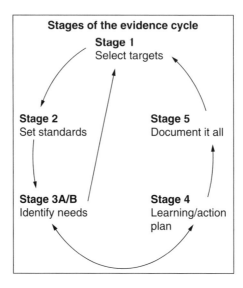

Stages of the evidence cycle

Stage 1
Select targets

Stage 2
Set standards

Stage 5
Document it all

Stage 3A/B
Identify needs

Stage 4
Learning/action plan

Case study 9.5

When you find yourself explaining lumbar X-ray results to two patients in the same surgery, you realise that you need to look into the frequency with which you and other GPs are organising X-rays for patients with back pain. One of these patients had previously seen a GP locum with their severe back pain of three days. One patient was yours and you had succumbed to the patient's pressure to organise an X-ray after their sciatic pain had persisted for two weeks, even though you knew it was not warranted clinically.

This is just an example. Keep your task simple. You could choose three or four cycles of evidence to demonstrate your competence as a GP each year.

Stage 1: Select your aspirations for good practice

The excellent GP:

- uses investigations when they will help the management of the condition
- gives patients the information they need about their problem, in a way they can understand.

Stage 2: Set the standards for your outcomes

> Outcomes might include:
>
> - the way learning is applied
> - a learnt skill
> - a protocol
> - a strategy that is implemented
> - meeting recommended standards.

- Ordering of lumbar–sacral X-rays for simple backache conforms to best practice.

Stage 3A: Identify your learning needs

- Undertake an audit of all lumbar–sacral X-rays over a six-month period ordered by you and others in the practice team. Compare the indications with the best practice guidance.[5,7,10]
- Consider the occasion when you 'gave in' to a patient's pressure and organised an investigation against your better judgement as a significant event. Analyse the circumstances and factors leading up to the event and think out how you might act differently in a similar situation in future. Discuss with a colleague whether they have any tips for you on being more assertive when it is in a patient's best interest to be so.

Stage 3B: Identify your service needs

> Any of the needs assessment exercises in 3A may also reveal service needs.

- Examine the medical notes of the last 10 patients for whom you or another GP organised a lumbar–sacral X-ray. Were there any 'red flag' features (*see* page 143) for which you should have referred the patient rather than arranging an X-ray in general practice? Is there any evidence that you/ other GPs put the patient(s) at risk by delaying referral?

- Draw up a map of the service providers relevant to the treatment of back pain in the NHS and private sector. Consider whether you know what their professional qualifications are, and if not obtain that information, before making any further referrals. Reflect on their expertise and find out from the PCO to whom you can refer. Determine whether there are gaps in services you can provide for patients and what you can do about it.

Stage 4: Make and carry out a learning and action plan

- Read up on best practice about the place of X-rays in managing simple backache.
- Attend communications skills workshops to hone your skills, especially in resisting inappropriate patient pressure for treatments or investigations.

Stage 5: Document your learning, competence, performance and standards of service delivery

- Include a copy of best practice in the ordering of lumbar–sacral X-rays for simple backache.
- Include your certificate of attendance at the communication skills workshops.
- Have a copy of the map of alternative service providers for treatment of back pain from a range of: physiotherapists, chiropractors, osteopaths, masseurs, Pilates practitioners, specialists in the Alexander technique, acupuncturists, orthopaedic consultants, etc.

Case study 9.5 continued

Both lumbar–sacral X-rays were normal. After undertaking the cycle of learning above and gathering the evidence, you present the information about best practice to your GP colleagues at a clinical update meeting. They have all been feeling uneasy about ordering unnecessary lumbar–sacral X-rays, and resolve with you to stick to the guidelines and remind each other if they slip back into their old habits.

References

1   Godlee F (2003) *Clinical Evidence Concise*. **Issue 10**. BMJ Publishing Group, London. www.clinicalevidence.com

2   van Tulder M and Koes B (2004) Low back pain and sciatica (chronic). *Clinical Evidence Concise*. **Issue 11**: 289–91.

3   Clinical Standards Advisory Group (1994) *Back Pain*. The Stationery Office, London.

4   Pengel L, Herbert RD, Maher CG *et al.* (2003) Acute low back pain: systematic review of its prognosis. *British Medical Journal*. **327**: 323–5.

5   National Institute for Clinical Excellence (NICE) (2004) Referral advice for acute low back pain. www.nice.org.uk

6   Car J and Sheikh A (2003) Acute low back pain. 10-minute consultation. *British Medical Journal*. **327**: 541.

7   Waddell G, McIntosh A, Hutchinson A *et al.* (1999) Low back pain evidence review. Royal College of General Practitioners, London.

8   Foord-Kelcey G (ed.) (2004) *Guidelines*. **23**: 338–9. www.eguidelines.co.uk

9   Chambers R, Hawksley B, Smith G *et al.* (2001) *Back Pain Matters in Primary Care*. Radcliffe Medical Press, Oxford.

10 Royal College of Radiologists (1998) *Making the Best Use of a Department of Clinical Radiology*. Royal College of Radiologists, London.

11 Woodman T (2004) *Doctor*. **15 January**: 22.

12 Moore A, Edwards J, Barden J *et al.* (eds) *Bandolier's Little Book of Pain*. Oxford University Press, Oxford.

13 Andersson G (1999) Epidemiological features of chronic low-back pain. *The Lancet*. **354**: 581–5.

14 Clinical Standards Advisory Group (1994) *Epidemiology Review: the epidemiology and cost of back pain*. The Stationery Office, London.

15 *Acute Musculoskeletal Pain: evidence-based management*. www.uq.edu.au/health/msp

16 Faculty of Occupational Medicine (2000) *Guidelines for the Management of Low Back Pain at Work*. Faculty of Occupational Medicine, London.

17 www.jr2.ox.ac.uk/bandolier/booth/booths/altmed.html

18 Developing patient partnerships www.dpp.org.uk

10

Palliative care

Case study 10.1

Dr Jolly, your GP registrar, brings some difficult cases to a tutorial with you. The common theme is that the patients are being cared for at home with an illness from which they are not expected to recover. He is finding it difficult to cope with his own feelings and with the team working necessary for the control of symptoms. He comments that he feels like a spare part, just writing out prescriptions suggested by the hospital specialist or by the palliative care nurse.

What issues you should cover

Palliative care is the support of people who are suffering from an illness from which no cure can be anticipated. Where possible, palliative care is delivered where the person wants to be. Usually it can be provided in a combination of:

- the person's own home
- a hospice
- a hospital
- a nursing home.

Family, relatives and friends are usually the main carers. Professional help comes from a team and is not just concerned with the relief of symptoms in people suffering from cancer, although it is often thought of in this narrow sense. The aim of palliative care is to maximise the quality of the person's life. Physical, emotional, social and spiritual needs may need attention. Meeting the individual needs of the person being cared for, and the caregivers, is a team effort that co-ordinates and delivers a range of services (*see* Figure 10.1).

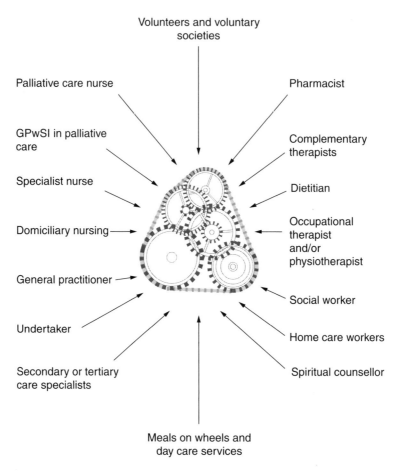

Figure 10.1: Some team members in palliative care.

Consider how information can be transferred from one carer to another. The individual being looked after, or his/her main carer, may not have the skills or knowledge to pass on details to others in the team of treatment or arrangements being made. Some patients and their carers like to keep a personal record of what is happening and what needs to be done. In most cases, the care plan and nursing notes, kept with the patient, are the best record of what treatment and plans are being made. Dr Jolly should make a point of reading these and recording (and signing legibly) any changes or arrangements he makes. These records can be invaluable if a stranger has to be involved – perhaps in an emergency at night when a different district nurse or doctor attends.

Treat each person as an individual

To understand the needs of another person, Dr Jolly must set aside his own beliefs or philosophy. Some concept of basic tenets of other cultures and religions will help him, but he must resist the urge to categorise patients. He has to find out about the expectations, values and beliefs of the person before him and what emotional, spiritual and practical support is available. Different cultures and religions have varying degrees of adherence and influence among communities. Sometimes there are different practices depending upon the country of origin of the individual or that of their family. As always, it is important to ask the person and those close to the sufferer. Anxiety, fear and hopelessness will make all other symptoms worse and less easy to manage, so the first task is to start from the standpoint of the sufferer and their carers, and help them to make some sense of what is happening. Giving information or helping people find the information they need, at a suitable pace, is a skill to be learnt. Knowing where to look for information can be the first step. Charitable organisations and patient groups can be immensely supportive, and an accessible website giving links to many other sources of help and guidance can be a useful resource for many patients, carers and professionals.[1]

Meetings with the patient and the carers to discuss what is needed, and whether the expectations for continuing help at home are being met, help to keep everyone on course for the smooth running of care. Regrettably, the lack of resources may mean that someone cannot be cared for at home as they wish, because of lack of, or delays in, sorting out benefits, equipment (such as hoists, bath aids, wheelchairs), or people who can help. The recommendations for a modern service for people with cancer,[2] and the various guidelines for people with cancer from NICE that are in preparation for 2004,[3] may help Dr Jolly know what the standard of service should be.

Dr Jolly may find that referral to a palliative care nurse has already been made by someone at the hospital before discharge home. If not, he may have to broach the subject himself and explore sensitively how someone would accept such referral. Many people believe that referral to a hospice, or for assessment by the community palliative care nurse, means that they are about to die. It is important to emphasise the support and specialist knowledge about relief of symptoms, provision of benefits, equipment and access to voluntary and professional help that the palliative care service can provide. After a referral, a community-based specialist nurse, usually a Macmillan nurse if the patient has cancer, will assess the whole situation.[4] Macmillan Cancer Relief helps provide expert care and practical support. They fund specialist Macmillan nurses, doctors and other health professionals and provide cancer care centres and hospices. They provide a range of information and support services, including the Macmillan CancerLine (the telephone helpline), useful publications and local cancer information centres.[4] They support local self-help groups and advise on, and sometimes give, financial support. They liaise with other professionals such as physiotherapists, occupational therapists and complementary therapists to provide the most appropriate care for the patient.

Macmillan nurses usually act in an advisory capacity but Marie Curie nurses are available in some areas to provide free nursing care. Marie Curie nurses now care for almost half of all cancer patients who die at home in the UK. They work through the night or during the day to provide one-on-one care for the patient and provide practical and emotional support for families at what can be an exhausting time.[1] In other areas, district nurse services, stretched at the best of times, have to be supplemented by volunteers, relatives or paid agency nurses.

If nursing care is not required, social services are asked to carry out a needs assessment and put into place means tested assistance, such as home care or meals on wheels. A social worker will also be able to help with applications for benefits. Dr Jolly may be asked to complete a 'DS1500'. The DS1500 is a form designed to speed up the payment of the Disability Living Allowance, Attendance Allowance or Incapacity Benefit. It is usually issued under special rules, after prior request by the patient or their carer, or at the suggestion of any primary care team member. The GP or a hospital consultant can complete the DS1500. It is usually issued when the patient is considered to be approaching the terminal stage of their disease. In Social Security law, a patient is terminally ill if they are suffering from a progressive disease and are not expected to live longer than six months. The timing is, of course, very difficult to judge, but the decision to issue is one for the clinician involved, who would then be able to justify their decision.

A GPwSI in palliative care (*see* Box 10.1) may be available for additional help and advice, and would provide an expert resource for Dr Jolly.

Box 10.1:   Role of a GPwSI in palliative care[5]

Core activities

Likely to work in one or more of:

- hospice or palliative care inpatient unit
- community-based palliative care team
- general practice with strong links with the above.

Clinical activities

May include:

- home visits and telephone advice service
- medical assessment, diagnosis and management planning
- advice on symptom control for advanced malignant and non-malignant disease

- ability to refer appropriately to other medical and non-medical agencies, including pain anaesthetist, counsellor or psychologist, and complementary therapies
- provision of care to patients in a hospice or other outpatient or inpatient setting
- provision of additional clinical services, such pleural drainage, paracentesis, drug or fluid infusion, blood transfusion, etc.

Education and liaison

- With other team members, develop and support the delivery of appropriate teaching for PCO clinicians.

Leadership and service development

- Support the development of good palliative care services in primary care.
- Integrate the primary care services with local specialist services.
- Develop practice-based cancer registers.
- Develop shared care.
- Take a lead role for clinical governance in palliative care within the PCO.

They may also be facilitators in palliative care set up and funded by the Macmillan Cancer Relief Fund.[6]

If the patient has another condition such as chronic obstructive pulmonary disease, Dr Jolly may need to find out how to contact relevant support services. The genitourinary medicine department usually organises the relevant specialist services for patients with acquired immunodeficiency syndrome (AIDS). Outreach specialist nurses may be available for particular conditions, but availability tends to be very variable from area to area. In a few areas, there is a common care pathway for any palliative care, but it is more common for it to be fragmented between departments and organisations. A practice resource list can help patients, carers and health professionals to contact the relevant sources of care and support.

Relief of symptoms

Dr Jolly should look at any previously prescribed medication to see if it is still relevant. It is often forgotten that medication may be prescribed to prevent events happening in the future e.g. treatment for hypertension, or to reduce cholesterol levels, which becomes irrelevant and unnecessary when the life expectancy is short. Previously prescribed medication may be contraindicated with the changes in treatment now required.

Pain

Dr Jolly should remember that not all pain is related to the primary condition – it may be secondary to the treatment – e.g. constipation due to opiates, gout precipitated by diuretics, or scar tissue after radiotherapy. It may be coincidental such as with migraine or osteoarthritis. Any perception of pain will be influenced by fear, loneliness, boredom, depression, previous experience of ill-health and individual attitudes.

Cancer pain is continuous, so it should be treated all the time, not just when it emerges. He should discuss the nature of chronic pain with patients who often believe that chronic pain is the same as acute pain only present all the time. Explain that acute pain is a danger signal that something is wrong. Chronic pain tells you that something has been wrong in the past and the nerves have become used to passing that signal onto the brain. Many people are unwilling to take adequate pain relief for chronic pain because they think they will not be able to receive acute pain warning signals. They need to be aware that they can relieve chronic pain with analgesics but still be able to feel the acute pain of, for example, cutting themselves on the edge of tin, or pulling a muscle during over-exertion. Beliefs about how chronic pain happens often lead people into inactivity. They avoid anything that might cause the pain in the short term instead of increasing their activity to improve muscle strength and co-ordination and stretch tight scar tissue to decrease the pain in the long term. Taking enough pain relief to prevent the emergence of pain, that is, prophylactically and not just in response to pain, reduces the passage of the pain messages along the nerves and helps to prevent the nerves becoming 'accustomed to passing that message'. Established pain leads to structural and neurochemical changes in the central nervous system that consolidate the pattern of pain. Taking enough pain relief also permits the graduated and frequent activity that improves chronic pain.

Cancer-related pain may be:

- soft-tissue or visceral pain and respond to paracetamol and opiates
- bone pain that can respond partially to paracetamol and opiates, or to NSAIDs, or be relieved by radiotherapy
- nerve-affected or nerve-mediated requiring drugs that act on the nervous system
- related to the impact of a cancer on adjacent tissues, e.g. in raised intracranial pressure or abdominal masses.

Most people in the UK prefer oral medications but consider with patients what would suit them best. There is increasing acceptance of transdermal application via a skin patch, although it may take some time to initially establish the right dose by titration. Some patients prefer suppositories if they have nausea or disturbed nights, because of break-through pain after shorter-acting oral medication. Paracetamol and opiates are generally used in a 'ladder' (*see* Box 10.2), increasing the dose of opiates until the pain is under control. Opiates also suppress cough and relieve breathlessness. Psychological techniques, such as cognitive therapy, can help patients to learn to manage their pain better and other techniques such as self-hypnosis or acupuncture may be helpful for some individuals.

Box 10.2: Analgesic ladder

Start here:
Non-opiate e.g. paracetamol
↓

Weak opiate e.g. codeine plus paracetamol: add medication to prevent constipation as soon as an opiate is added
↓

Strong opiate e.g. morphine plus non-opioid or fentanyl patch (*see British National Formulary*[7] for equivalent strength to morphine), e.g.:

- start with oral morphine 10 mg 4 hourly (i.e. six times a day)
- increase by a third to half every 3–5 days according to response
- transfer to the same dose of slow release morphine every 12 h (or a patch), with standard release morphine available for break-through pain or increases as required.

Other medications that can help to control pain are listed in Table 10.1 (overleaf).

Dr Jolly should anticipate the common problems when introducing opiates. A stimulant laxative should be added as soon as an opiate is started and the dose increased when the opiate strength is increased. A softening or bulking agent alone is rarely successful. Sleepiness is usual when starting each dose increment and then wears off. Nausea is also common (*see* Table 10.2). Other problems can include a dry mouth, itching, sweating, hallucinations and myoclonic jerks. Although tolerance may occur, increases in dose are usually required for advancing disease. Always look at other causes for pain breakthrough.

Constipation

Doctors often have poor knowledge about constipation. Exclude constipation as the cause of agitation and distress before adding in other drugs. Clinical examination should include abdominal and rectal examination. Never forget that uncontrolled diarrhoea may be overflow liquid finding its way past a valve-like effect of hard faeces. A good first choice for the prevention of opiate induced or inactivity constipation is a combination of a stimulant laxative

Table 10.1: Additional medication to control non-opiate sensitive pain[8]

Type of pain	Medication	Considerations
Bone pain Pleuritic pain Soft tissue infiltration	Non-steroidal anti-inflammatory drugs (NSAIDs) Consider radiotherapy	Avoid NSAIDs if a previous history of gastrointestinal ulceration. Selective Cox II inhibitors reduce but do not completely avoid risks of gastrointestinal upset and damage. NSAIDs can be given with a proton pump inhibitor e.g. lansoprozole
Raised intracranial pressure Enlarged liver or spleen Enlarging tumours	Steroids Consider radiotherapy	Dexametasone usually used (2 mg dexametasone = 15 mg prednisolone) Gastroprotection also required as for NSAIDs
Nerve related pain e.g. shooting, stabbing or burning	Amitriptyline Carbamazepine, gabapentin	Used in lower doses than for depression, start low and increase to reduce sedation and dry mouth Higher dose use may be limited by the side-effects
Root pain	Steroids, trancutaneous electrical nerve stimulation (TENS machine), consider nerve block	A loan of a TENS machine can usually be arranged
Muscle spasm	Diazepam Baclofen	May cause sedation but can also relieve anxiety Increase dose slowly to avoid sedation and muscle hypotonia
Tenesmus	As for nerve related pain Chlorpromazine Nifedipine	 Sedation a problem but useful if restlessness also present Increase dose slowly to avoid flushing

together with a softening agent, e.g. co-danthrusate, co-danthramer, or senna with lactulose.[8] High doses of lactulose can cause flatulence and abdominal cramps. Relatively high doses of laxative may be needed. Tailor your treatment of existing constipation according to your clinical findings:

* rectum full of hard faeces: lubricate with glycerin suppositories or an oil enema, then use a stimulant laxative with or without a softener
* rectum full of soft faeces: use a stimulant laxative which will take about 10 hours to work

- rectum still full after the above treatment: manual evacuation, perhaps with sedation or an anxiolytic
- rectum empty: consider if obstruction is present or high constipation
- loaded colon with colic: start a softener, e.g. docusate
- loaded colon without colic: try a stimulant laxative.

Nausea and/or vomiting

Constipation may be accompanied by nausea or nausea may be present alone with or without vomiting. Useful medications are listed in Table 10.2.

Using drugs in a syringe driver

A syringe driver is a useful alternative if gastric symptoms are a persistent problem despite medication, or if the patient prefers not to have medication orally. Diamorphine is the opiate of choice for subcutaneous infusion because of its high solubility. It also helps with breathlessness. Divide the dose of morphine by three to convert from morphine to diamorphine. Other drugs can be added to the syringe driver (*see* Table 10.2). Midazolam can be added to control restlessness, myoclonic jerks or as an anticonvulsant if required. The syringe driver needs to be checked regularly for irritation at the injection site, crystallisation of the drugs, leakage, correct volume remaining and that the battery is not exhausted. Drugs used in the syringe driver may be used outside their product licence, so keep meticulous records. It is good practice to use as few drugs as possible in the syringe driver, usually only one or two, as data on compatibility are sparse. Water for injection is usually used as the diluent, as physiological saline may cause precipitation when more than one drug is used.[7]

Complementary therapies[9]

Acupuncture is often used successfully for both pain relief and treatment of nausea. Surveys of the available scientific research into acupuncture suggest that it is definitely an effective treatment for nausea caused by chemotherapy when treating cancer.[9]

Aromatherapy may help with relaxation and feelings of improved well-being. Particularly when combined with massage, the close physical contact and the relationship with a therapist can help to increase people's sense of being cared for. Caution is required where essential oils are used that may affect skin that is already sensitive following radiotherapy.

Hypnotherapy may be used as an adjunct to other therapy and has been shown to ameliorate some psychological and medical conditions. It can be

Table 10.2: Some drugs for nausea and vomiting.[8] Consult the *British National Formulary*[7] for others less commonly used

Drug and action	Other indications	Characteristics	Cautions
Metoclopropamide* Increases peristalsis in upper gut Dopamine antagonist		Oral tablets or liquid Intramuscular injection	Extrapyramidal effects especially in children or young people
Domperidone Increases peristalsis in upper gut Dopamine antagonist		Oral tablets or liquid Suppositories	Less likely to cause dystonia
Cyclizine* Acts on vestibular and vomiting centres	Vertigo	Oral tablets Intramuscular, intravenous injection	Drowsiness Caution in severe heart failure
Haloperidol* Blocks dopamine receptors at chemoreceptor trigger zone	Hiccups Psychotic symptoms Agitation	Oral tablets Intramuscular, intravenous injection	Dry mouth, hypotension, extrapyramidal symptoms
Levomeprazine* Blocks dopamine and serotonin receptors, also acts at vestibular and vomiting centres	Psychotic symptoms Adjunct for pain Agitation	Oral tablets Intramuscular, intravenous injection	Postural hypotension Sedation
Ondansetron* **Granisetron** Blocks 5-HT$_3$ receptors	Especially for nausea and vomiting induced by chemotherapy	Oral tablets Intramuscular, intravenous injection Ondansetron also in suppositories	Constipation, flushing and rash
Dexametasone* Reduces inflammatory oedema, central and peripheral anti-emetic effects	Pain relief	Oral tablets Intramuscular, intravenous injection	Steroid side-effects
Hyoscine hydrobromide* Reduces gastrointestinal secretions and motility	Excessive respiratory secretions Motion sickness	Oral tablets, patch, intramuscular injection	Closed angle glaucoma, urinary retention, gastrointestinal obstruction
Octreotide * **Lanreotide*** Reduces gastrointestinal secretions and motility	Relief of symptoms from neuroendocrine tumours Variceal bleeding	Subcutaneous injection	Affects diabetic control

* Also useful in a syringe driver as a subcutaneous infusion used together with therapies such as cognitive behavioural therapy to enable patients to view their illness in a less negative or catastrophic way.[9]

Over-the-counter herbal therapies should not be taken. Always ask about any herbal remedies or supplements as they may be contraindicated unless prescribed by a medical herbalist with full knowledge of the conventional medication being taken.[10] Many herbal remedies interact with medication e.g. St John's Wort with medication for AIDS or ginger with warfarin. Some may be contraindicated in certain cancers, e.g. echinacea in lymphoma.[11]

Other complementary therapies e.g. Reiki, head massage, spiritual healing, may also be offered by the local hospice or obtained elsewhere by patients and their carers. Benefits of improved symptom control, quality of life and patient satisfaction have been demonstrated, but various questions remain. The quality of evidence for many of these therapies is poor and it is not known if the specific techniques are as important as their shared 'holistic' context. The lack of evidence about the way in which therapies work also obscures any possible unwanted effects. Although many of the therapies make patients feel better, claims for improvements to survival from cancer may give false hope.[9]

Dry mouth

A dry mouth is a distressing and frequent problem. Good mouth care, sucking ice or pineapple chunks or artificial saliva may help. Take swabs for thrush if suspected – it may just look red and shiny, not with the classic white patches – and if confirmed, treat with antifungal preparations, e.g. nystatin, miconazole or amphotericin.[7] Bacterial or viral infections should be treated, and malignant ulcers are often infected with anaerobic bacteria causing a foul smell. Treat anaerobic infections with metronidazole orally, rectally or as a gel.[7]

Distress

Perhaps the most important treatment is for people to spend time with the patient – to appreciate with the patient what life was like before, to acknowledge the person that remains despite the illness and disability, and to show care for the patient and the carers, discussing what would help to make life more comfortable or bearable. Sometimes it is more important for patients to be able to talk than to have drug treatment for their symptoms. Some patients become more agitated and distressed when they do not feel in control of their mental functions because of inappropriate sedation.

Giving bad news is a skill that is difficult to acquire.[12] Always check with patients that what they have heard you say is what you mean – health professionals often use words that patients do not understand, even when they are trying to explain things clearly. Also, consider the response of the individual – it will always be different from the last person you talked to about similar bad news. Go at the pace of the patient and always establish what they already know, or think they know, before giving any more information. Health professionals have to talk, not just about the illness, but also about the treatments, the need for tests, and about the uncertainty of the future. Such details may need to be repeated because of the difficulties in taking in information when emotionally upset. Anger, guilt and blame are common reactions people have to bad news. These emotions need understanding and discussion, so that the emotion is not directed towards inappropriate targets, such as blaming themselves, health professionals or their god.

Dr Jolly will have his own feelings to cope with as well. Identification with the emotions of the patient and carers and feelings of failure are common. Denial is a common mechanism for coping, and may lead to collusion not to mention the seriousness of the condition. Denial is rarely complete and Dr Jolly can use the same open-ended questions that he employs in his everyday consultations, e.g. 'I wonder how it looks to you?' Dr Jolly may want to consider attending a course to help him with this type of problem,[12] or just generally improve his communication skills. He might look at the competencies that a GPwSI is expected to have (*see* Box 10.3), so that he has some goals at which to aim.

Box 10.3:   Core competencies recommended for a GPwSI in palliative care[13]

Generalist

- Good communication skills, including breaking bad news, dealing with conflict and denial, communication with families, dealing with the practicalities of death and bereavement
- Clear understanding of palliative care and symptom control
- Ability to diagnose common complications of advanced cancer and non-malignant disease

Specialist

- Excellent multidisciplinary team-working skills, with a clear understanding of the roles of the other members of the team
- Good leadership skills
- Ability to establish a practice-based palliative care register and use it for call, recall, audit and outcome
- If appropriate, an ability to perform a number of practical procedures, e.g. chest drainage

---

Emergencies

Dr Jolly should think about how to avoid emergencies, especially as these often result in a patient having an otherwise avoidable hospital admission. These include:

- hypercalcaemia
- bone fractures
- superior vena caval obstruction
- spinal cord compression
- epileptic seizures
- haemorrhage.

Hypercalcaemia occurs in 40–50% of people with multiple myeloma and breast cancer, less often in other cancers.[8] Treatment of hypercalcaemia can markedly improve the patient's symptoms even when the disease is advanced. In mild hypercalaemia, patients have symptoms of nausea, anorexia and vomiting, with thirst, polyuria and constipation – non-specific symptoms common in terminal care – so he needs to think about it and be prepared to check serum calcium. More severe symptoms include dehydration, drowsiness, confusion and coma, and cardiac arrhythmias. The corrected calcium level is calculated with the value for serum albumin, so this also needs to be checked, together with urea and electrolytes in case an intravenous infusion is required. Saline for rehydration may be followed by a biphosphonate infusion.[8] Treatment with biphosphonates usually corrects the serum calcium in 80% of patients within a week. Treatment of the underlying cancer may prevent recurrence, but if not, oral biphosphonates or infusions every three weeks may be needed.

Bone fractures may be prevented by oral biphosphonates, but they may still occur in osteoporosis, metastatic osteolytic deposits or secondary to trauma. Appropriate treatment depends on the general state of the patient but may include fixation or radiotherapy.

The symptoms of obstruction of the vena cava are very frightening, with severe breathlessness and a sensation of drowning. Other symptoms include swelling of the face, especially around the eyes, neck and arms. The patient may complain of visual changes, headache, dizziness and fainting. Give immediate treatment with small doses of opiates e.g. 5 mg every four hours if not already receiving an opiate, with or without diazepam. High-dose corticosteroids (dexametasone 16 mg/day) can usually be reduced after the first five days, and referral for radiotherapy discussed.

Spinal cord compression may be gradual and difficult to spot in its early stages. Weakness of the legs is often attributed to the general state of debility, and urinary or bowel problems to the medication. Dr Jolly needs to think of spinal cord compression in any patient with cancer who complains of back pain, especially if any neurological signs are also present. A magnetic resonance scan can localise any areas of compression and allow targeted radiotherapy.

A patient who has a brain tumour or secondary deposits may need an anticonvulsant. If oral medication is discontinued, Dr Jolly should anticipate the need for alternative delivery of anticonvulsant medication e.g. midazolam 30 mg/24 h via a syringe driver, or rectal diazepam (10 mg).

If the patient is coughing up blood, Dr Jolly needs to establish where the bleeding originates – the chest, nose, upper respiratory tract or even the GI tract. Bleeding may need to be controlled by radiotherapy or laser therapy. In the last few hours of life, haemoptysis, haematemesis or erosion of a major blood vessel may cause distressing loss of blood. He should make sure that medication is available so that an injection (intravenously if there is circulatory shut-down) of an opiate and diazepam can help to reduce awareness and fear in the patient. Anticipation and preparation help to reduce the distress of carers, and the use of green or dark-coloured towels reduces the visual impact.

Case study 10.1 continued

After the tutorial, Dr Jolly draws up a plan to meet some of his learning needs. In the process of helping him meet some of these from the practice resources and elsewhere, you learn quite a bit as well! He begins to feel more competent and able to be proactive in some suggestions for meeting the needs of patients who require palliative care. He finds talking to the palliative care nurse helps him to understand how he might learn to cope with his emotional responses, and is relieved to find that that other professionals suffer from doubts and difficulties as well.

Collecting data to demonstrate your learning, competence, performance and standards of service delivery

Example cycle of evidence 10.1

- Focus: relationships with patients
- Other relevant foci: clinical care; working with colleagues

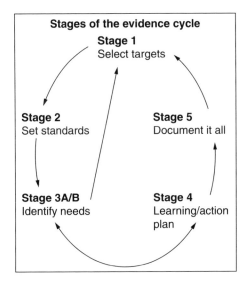

Case study 10.2

Mrs Ovum had been admitted to hospital urgently with a large pleural effusion and after many tests disseminated ovarian cancer had been diagnosed. She was discharged home after a course of chemotherapy and has asked for a home visit. When you arrive her mother lets you in and whispers to you in the hallway: 'She doesn't know what is wrong with her. She thinks she has had treatment for an ovarian cyst'. Her husband is also there, while her father has taken the children out for a while. Mrs Ovum asks you to explain what she has had done at the hospital and says that she cannot understand why she feels so tired. You can tell by the non-verbal signals and anxious looks of her relatives that you could easily say the wrong thing.

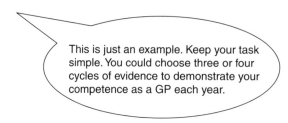

Stage 1: Select your aspirations for good practice

The excellent GP:

- is up to date with developments in clinical practice and regularly reviews his or her knowledge and performance
- is guided by the patient in revealing information about the amount and nature of information that he/she wishes to have.

Stage 2: Set the standards for your outcomes

Outcomes might include:

- the way learning is applied
- a learnt skill
- a protocol
- a strategy that is implemented
- meeting recommended standards.

- A comprehensive source of information about terminal conditions is available to members of the practice team.
- Team members caring for someone who is terminally ill communicate to each other their actions and the information given to patients.

Stage 3A: Identify your learning needs

- Establish whether you know how to find information about specific cancer treatments or patient support organisations.
- Self-assess how much you know about how and what to tell patients about their terminal condition.
- Reflect on how you manage the conflict between telling the truth and protecting patients from psychological distress.

Stage 3B: Identify your service needs

Any of the needs assessment exercises in 3A may also reveal service needs.

- Audit the records of three patients with terminal conditions to identify any gaps in communication between team members.
- Review the length of time patients with terminal conditions are waiting for treatment by others or for equipment e.g. by an occupational therapist, for a commode, or for a TENS machine, and the waiting time for an initial appointment with a palliative care nurse. Consider what you might have done to speed any of these processes, including supplying evidence to your PCO to influence the commissioning process.

Stage 4: Make and carry out a learning and action plan

- Read information about investigations into how patients are told about a terminal diagnosis.[12,14]
- Look up information about ovarian cancer so that you know enough to discuss it if necessary.[15]
- Attend a workshop examining the ethical and practical dilemmas of managing patients with terminal illnesses.
- Run an educational session at the practice for other GPs, practice nurses, attached physiotherapist, district nurses, the palliative care nurse and any others with an interest, to share patients' views and the results of your audit on the difficulties and gaps in communication. Present the draft treatment policy for discussion, before accepting it as a practice team.
- Discuss how the agreed treatment policy can be implemented with key people in the practice team and decide what shortfalls there are in terms of resources (e.g. availability of equipment or therapy or over-long referral routes) and liaise with the PCO about unmet needs. Find out if there is a GPwSI whose expertise can be used.[13]

Stage 5: Document your learning, competence, performance and standards of service delivery

- Your reflective diary comments about how you manage the conflict between telling the truth and protecting patients from psychological distress and what you can put into practice from the workshop.
- Keep notes on best practice and ovarian cancer from your information search.

- Include a copy of the agreed practice policy for communication between team members caring for someone who is receiving palliative care.
- Include a copy of the letter to the PCO detailing shortfalls in provision for palliative care.
- Include the letter of thanks you receive from Mrs Ovum's mother for your help.

Case study 10.2 continued

You ask Mrs Ovum what she knows about her condition. She says that she had a large ovarian cyst that was causing pressure on her lungs and she has had chemotherapy to shrink the cyst, as it could not be removed. You talk about the side-effects of chemotherapy and how tired that can make someone feel. She seems happier at this information and you ask her to write down any questions she thinks of after your visit and you can discuss them next time. You resolve to look up information about ovarian cancer so that you are better prepared if Mrs Ovum asks you outright about ovarian cancer.[1,15] On the way out, her mother tries to impress on you that you must not tell Mrs Ovum that she has cancer. You acknowledge and comfort her about her own distress about her daughter's illness. You tell her that many patients with cancer know that they have it, but do not want to discuss it. You say to Mrs Ovum's mother that you will be guided by what Mrs Ovum wants to talk about.

Over the next few weeks, it emerges that Mrs Ovum is aware of her diagnosis but has been trying to hide this from her mother. Many tears are shed when the two of them are able to talk more openly about the future.

Example cycle of evidence 10.2

- Focus: if things go wrong
- Other relevant focus: keeping good records

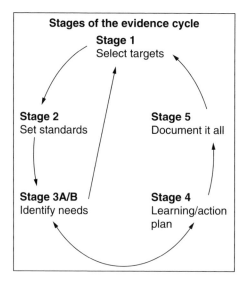

Stages of the evidence cycle

Stage 1
Select targets

Stage 2
Set standards

Stage 5
Document it all

Stage 3A/B
Identify needs

Stage 4
Learning/action
plan

Case study 10.3

You receive a message to ring the coroner about Mr Blow. The coroner's officer tells you that the Registrar of Births, Deaths and Marriages has said that she has the death certificate for Mr Blow but the daughter had told her that her father was a miner and was receiving disablement benefit. You had given the cause of death as bronchial carcinoma with chronic obstructive airways disease as a secondary cause. The coroner's officer reminds you that if pneumoconiosis is a possible underlying cause, the death should be referred to the coroner, and an inquest may need to be held to determine if an industrial disease is present. You have only been attending Mr Blow in the last six months since he moved into his daughter's house but had visited many times during his terminal illness. You are upset to find that you had not recorded that he had been a miner, so had not thought of the implications when you issued the death certificate for an expected death.

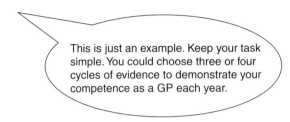

This is just an example. Keep your task simple. You could choose three or four cycles of evidence to demonstrate your competence as a GP each year.

Stage 1: Select your aspirations for good practice

The excellent GP:

- contacts the patient or relative soon after it is apparent that a mistake has occurred
- tells the patient or relative what has happened and how it can be put right
- co-operates with any investigation arising from a complaint.

Stage 2: Set the standards for your outcomes

Outcomes might include:

- the way learning is applied
- a learnt skill
- a protocol
- a strategy that is implemented
- meeting recommended standards.

- There is a record of how the practice team learns from a mistake to minimise a recurrence.
- A revised practice protocol is agreed for recording industrial or notifiable diseases.

Stage 3A: Identify your learning needs

- Undertake a significant event audit of Mr Blow's case with the team responsible for his terminal care.
- Discuss the process of dealing with a complaint with the practice manager and medical defence society, so that you know how to respond.

Stage 3B: Identify your service needs

> Any of the needs assessment exercises in 3A may also reveal service needs.

- Invite a coroner to talk to a meeting arranged for practices in your PCO, to identify those conditions that should be notified to the coroner.
- Audit 50 records of patients over the age of 65 years, to establish how many of them have a record of a potentially notifiable previous employment.
- Identify what resources are available in the practice for informing patients of diseases for which benefit payments may be payable.

Stage 4: Make and carry out a learning and action plan

- Read up about welfare rights implications of a diagnosis of pneumoconiosis and other industrial diseases, and make a resource file so that other team members can refer to it.[16,17]
- Work with the practice team to learn from the significant event audit of Mr Blow's case, and make an action plan to minimise recurrence. You might add a reminder to a diagnosis of chronic obstructive airways disease, carcinoma of the lung, deafness, or other possible notifiable diseases, to ensure that significant past employment is recorded on computer or paper-based medical records.
- Attend and record learning points from the talk given by the coroner.

Stage 5: Document your learning, competence, performance and standards of service delivery

- Keep notes of the significant event audit and subsequent action plan.
- Include a copy of the audit of patient records of how many of them have a record of a potentially notifiable previous employment, and the date to repeat the audit after implementation of the action plan.
- Include a list of the learning points from the talk given by the coroner.
- Include a copy of the resource document about the welfare rights implications of industrial diseases that is available on the practice computer or in the practice library.

> **Case study 10.3 continued**
> Mr Blow's daughter is pleased that you contacted her. You apologise for your lack of knowledge and for the mistake in not explaining to her that the death would need to be examined by the coroner because of the financial implications.

You are able to put her in touch with sources of help for ex-miners.[16] Later, when you see her again, she comments that she found this very helpful both for the practical advice and emotionally. You and the practice team become much more aware of the welfare rights issues involved in industrial diseases and are able to help several other patients apply for benefits that they did not know about.

Example cycle of evidence 10.3

- Focus: teaching and training
- Other relevant foci: relationships with patients; maintaining good medical practice

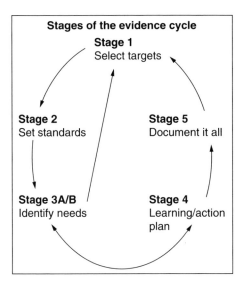

Stages of the evidence cycle

Stage 1
Select targets

Stage 2
Set standards

Stage 5
Document it all

Stage 3A/B
Identify needs

Stage 4
Learning/action plan

Case study 10.4

A medical student is sitting in your surgery when Mrs Rosary and her son, Kappa, attend. You are taken aback by the boy's appearance – an eleven-year-old wearing dark glasses, a baseball hat, and very large baggy clothes, with his hands stuffed in his pockets. You keep a non-committal expression but see the student make a face and roll his eyes up. Mrs Rosary tells you that their church is sponsoring Kappa to go to Lourdes. You had completely forgotten that seven months ago, one of your partners told you that Kappa had been diagnosed with leukaemia. He has not been seen by anyone in the surgery since, and Mrs Rosary tells you that they attend a distant teaching hospital frequently. There is very little recent information in his medical records about his progress. Mrs Rosary hands you a large packet of forms and asks if you will fill them in so that Kappa can go to Lourdes. You flick through them and see that they require details of his treatment and current state of health – and you have little idea about either. When they leave, the medical student says 'What a weird-looking kid!'.

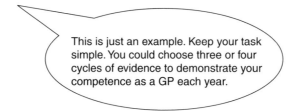

This is just an example. Keep your task simple. You could choose three or four cycles of evidence to demonstrate your competence as a GP each year.

Stage 1: Select your aspirations for good practice

The excellent GP:

- helps to educate other colleagues at all levels
- does not undermine the confidence of juniors or students
- treats patients with courtesy and consideration
- keeps his/her knowledge up to date.

Stage 2: Set the standards for your outcomes

Outcomes might include:

- the way learning is applied
- a learnt skill
- a protocol
- a strategy that is implemented
- meeting recommended standards.

- Demonstrate an active involvement in the training of another.
- Behave in a courteous way to patients and students.
- Demonstrate a willingness to find out information not readily available.
- An automatic practice-based review process for patients with a new diagnosis of cancer is in place.

Stage 3A: Identify your learning needs

- Gain peer review of your teaching skills – ask another trainer to peer review a tutorial with the medical student.
- Self-assess your awareness of the curriculum of the local medical school.
- Read the information supplied in the pack with the forms about going to Lourdes so that you are better informed about what is required.
- Feedback from trainees is good way to assess your teaching, although it may be difficult to avoid bias if feedback is not anonymised.
- Check whether you have the skills to guide the student to manage this type of consultation, and to show him how the patient might suffer if he is perceived to be judgemental.

Stage 3B: Identify your service needs

> Any of the needs assessment exercises in 3A may also reveal service needs.

- Undertake a force-field analysis with others in the practice team about the driving and restraining factors involved in teaching medical students.
- Discuss the lack of feedback from the teaching hospital at a practice meeting to determine whether this is a common problem and how to remedy the lack of information in future.
- Discuss why no one at the practice was aware of the lack of knowledge about Kappa's illness and how a practice register of patients with cancer might help with this.

Stage 4: Make and carry out a learning and action plan

- Attend a meeting of the medical school curriculum group and reflect what parts you can use for guiding your teaching.
- Obtain and read the feedback from the teaching hospital about Kappa's treatment and prognosis.
- Use this information as well as reading to prepare for a tutorial with the medical student about modern treatment for leukaemia and the role of faith healing.[18]
- Attend a 'Training the trainers' course, or if it is a while since you last went on a course, a refresher course may be a good idea.
- Reflect on the outcome of the force-field analysis with another GP or nurse teachers in the practice. Make a plan to boost the driving factors.

- Obtain advice from the PCO, from the GPwSI in palliative care if there is one, or from the educational lead, about how a practice register of patients with cancer might be utilised.

Stage 5: Document your learning, competence, performance and standards of service delivery

- Keep a record of your discussion with, and the feedback from, the medical student about leukaemia, professional conduct and faith healing.
- Record the information about the curriculum and how you will use it.
- Record the outcome of the force-field analysis.
- Record your notes about your new knowledge on leukaemia and about Lourdes.
- Keep a record of your notes on what you learnt on the trainers' course, with your certificate of attendance.
- Keep a record of your letter to the teaching hospital recording your disquiet at the lack of feedback and their reply, and send a copy to your PCO with the patient details anonymised in case this is a more widespread problem.
- Record how the practice register of patients with cancer will be set up and used, with reviews of newly diagnosed patients at six months to assess support needs and secondary care, to ensure that the practice can claim six quality points.

Case study 10.3 continued

In your discussion with the medical student, you guide him into acknowledging that Kappa may be hiding beneath his weird image to disguise his bald head, lack of eyebrows and thin frame following treatment. You have a useful discussion with the student about how health professionals should behave. Following your correspondence with the teaching hospital and your reading, you know a lot more about leukaemia and are able to give a tutorial with confidence. You contact Mrs Rosary to say that you have completed the forms from the information from the hospital, and Kappa does not need a medical. You wish them well for the pilgrimage.

Your partners are pleased that all the discussion has been worthwhile in improving the care of patients with cancer and ensuring that the practice can justify claiming the quality points for cancer care.

References

1 www.hospice-spc-council.org.uk/

2 NHS Modernisation Agency (2003) *Gold Standards Framework Project in Community Palliative Care.* Department of Health, London. www.modern.nhs.uk/cancer

3 www.nice.org.uk

4 www.macmillan.org.uk Telephone helpline: freephone +44 (0)808 808 2020; textphone +44 (0)808 808 0121 Monday to Friday 9 am–6 pm.

5 Department of Health (2003) *Guidelines for the Appointment of General Practitioners with Special Interests in the Delivery of Clinical Services: palliative care.* Department of Health, London.

6 Macmillan Cancer Relief Fund. www.macmillan.org.uk

7 Joint Formulary Committee (2003) *British National Formulary.* British Medical Association/Royal Pharmaceutical Society, London. www.bnf.org

8 Fallon M and O'Neill B (eds) (1998) *ABC of Palliative Care.* BMJ Books, London.

9 Tavares M (2003) *National Guidelines for the Use of Complementary Therapy.* The Prince of Wales's Foundation for Integrated Health, London, England. www.hospice-spc-council.org.uk/public/complementaryguidelines.pdf

10 Ernst E (2000) Herbal medicine: where is the evidence? *British Medical Journal.* **321:** 395–6.

11 Medicines Control Agency (2002) *Safety of Herbal Medicinal Products.* Department of Health, London. www.mca.gov.uk/ourwork/licensingmeds/herbalmeds/HerbalsSafetyReportJuly2002_Final.pdf

12 Fallowfield L and Jenkins V (2004) Communicating sad, bad and difficult news in medicine. *Lancet.* **363:** 312–19.

13 www.dh.gov.uk/assetRoot/04/06/83/75/04068375.pdf

14 Leliopoulo C, Wilkinson SM and Fellowes D (2001) *Does Truth Telling Improve Psychological Distress of Palliative Care Patients: a systematic review. Curie Palliative Care Research and Development Unit. 1–20.* Available from the Dare reviews at www.york.ac.uk/inst/crd

15 www.ovacome.org.uk

16 Coal Industry Social Welfare Organisation addresses of local offices and information from www.ciswo.org.uk

17 Industrial Injuries Disablement Benefit (diseases and deafness) www.jobcentreplus.gov.uk/cms.asp?Page=/Home/Customers/WorkingAgeBenefits

18 Greaves M (2002) Science, medicine, and the future: Childhood leukaemia: Clinical review. *British Medical Journal.* **324:** 283–7.

11

Good prescribing practice

Case study 11.1

Richard is the prescribing lead for his PCO. He really took on the role because none of the other GPs on the executive of the PCO would volunteer. Once he has taken on this lead role he realises that he should ensure that he and his partners are actually following best practice themselves, and determines to review prescribing in general and the practice repeat prescribing system in particular.

What issues you should cover

A repeat prescription is a 'prescription issued without a consultation'.[1] Good quality practice means producing an efficient repeat prescribing system that incorporates clinical feedback and regular monitoring. Best practice in repeat prescribing systems reduces the opportunities for prescription fraud as well as increasing the effectiveness of treatment regimes and patient safety.

Repeat prescribing accounts for a significant proportion of all medication prescribed. One study, reporting on 115 practices, found that repeat prescriptions were responsible for 75% of all items and 81% of prescribing costs; 48% of all registered patients received a repeat prescription at least once over a period of one year.[1] Another study of repeat prescribing found that there was no evidence of authorisation by a doctor in two-thirds of repeat prescriptions and that 72% of repeat prescriptions had not been reviewed in the previous 15 months.[2]

Best practice in generating a prescription

Whether the prescription is computer generated or handwritten, the drug name, strength, dose, frequency and quantity should all be clearly stated and written in ink, to lessen the likelihood of misinterpretations or mistakes by the dispenser, or patients altering the prescription contents. The quantities of any drug liable to abuse should be written in words and figures.

Where additions or corrections are made, the practitioner signing the prescription should initial or countersign against them. Ancillary staff who write, or are involved in the preparation of, repeat prescriptions should be appropriately trained in:

- the practice protocols for repeat prescribing
- what their responsibilities are
- the need for accuracy.[2]

Practice staff who use the practice computer to generate repeat prescriptions should have an individual password that can be used at a later date, to identify the member of staff who prepared the prescription for signing. Not all practice computers have this facility and it is recommended that all computer systems should be able to provide such audit trails. No one member of the practice staff should be entirely responsible for one part of the prescription-generating process. Involvement of more than one staff member aids informal checking of procedures and deters fraud.

Blank prescriptions should never be signed by a doctor and completed afterwards by either the doctor or a delegate.

When prescriptions are to be signed by GP registrars, assistants, locums or deputies, the name of the doctor printed at the bottom of the script will be that of the responsible GP principal.

Unused space should be cancelled out under the last drug by a computerised mechanism or the doctor deleting the space manually. The current issue of the *British National Formulary* describes good practices for computer-issued prescriptions and prescription writing and you should endeavour to adhere to these.[3]

Dealing with a request for a repeat prescription

General practices should have an agreed written protocol for generating repeat prescriptions. Prescriptions should only be repeated if authorised by a doctor or other practitioner who is qualified as a prescriber.[2] The repeat prescriptions process should be well advertised to patients on their registered list. The standards set out in the protocol for the time between receipt of request and production of prescription should allow adequate time for a good-quality repeat prescribing system to operate. Ancillary staff and GPs should adhere to the repeat prescribing protocol, rather than cutting corners or overriding the usual procedures when errors might be made.

It is good practice for the patient, or their representative who is independent of any person or organisation involved in the prescribing or dispensing process, to initiate the request for specific repeat medication. If the patient or representative is not involved in such a request, there may be opportunities for fraud. If pharmacists do request repeat prescriptions as well as provide a collection service, there is a professional requirement that they should retain in the pharmacy a signed declaration by the patient that it is their wish for medicines to be dispensed at that pharmacy. Box 11.1 summarises the key points in repeat prescribing practice.

Box 11.1:   Key points in best practice in repeat prescribing[1-6]

- The GP should retain an active involvement throughout the repeat prescribing process and should not delegate any entire part of the process to ancillary staff.
- The patient, or his/her representative who is independent of any contractor involved in prescribing or dispensing the prescription, should have an active role in requesting a repeat prescription, and not be bypassed by contractors, however well meaning.
- The practice must control its repeat prescribing system properly. The system must be programmed to obtain reports that reveal areas requiring closer attention and trigger patient reviews at appropriate time periods.
- Extra vigilance is required when prescribing for nursing and residential homes.
- Requests for repeat prescribing should not be initiated by pharmacies without involving patients or their carers.

Written requests for repeat medication are preferable to oral requests. Written requests are more likely to be accurately recorded, as many drugs sound similar. Written requests also reduce opportunities for fraud and misunderstandings. Computerised request forms, with desired items ticked by patients and submitted on a regular basis are preferable to handwritten *ad hoc* requests.

The person requesting a repeat prescription on behalf of another should be known to the patient, or be able to prove that they represent that patient.

Computerised request forms should indicate unambiguously that patients or their representatives should only tick items needed, and that those not ticked will not be deleted from the repeat prescription system.

GPs signing repeat prescriptions should be able to access the relevant patients' records easily to cross check the validity and appropriateness of the request.

A 28-day supply of a prescription is generally accepted as striking an optimal balance between patient convenience, good clinical practice and minimal drug wastage. It is good practice to prescribe a common number of days' treatments for each repeat prescribed item. There will be acceptable exceptions such as for oral contraception, hormone replacement therapy and a few other types of long-term medication, where items attract multiple prescription charges or need infrequent review.

The practice protocol should define the time intervals at which each type of repeat medication should be reviewed by a doctor, to make sure that the drugs are still appropriate and needed. A comprehensive review will usually only be possible if the patient or his/her records are reviewed individually. Best practice is where computerised systems are in place to trigger the necessity for a doctor's review at the required time, according to the practice protocol for that particular drug. The best computer systems have a 'lock out' facility where only the prescriber can override and extend the medication review period.

All repeat prescriptions issued should be recorded in the medical records whether paper or computer records.

Repeat prescriptions should be discontinued when their therapeutic effect has ceased. The practice system should be able to efficiently eliminate or change the dose of a specific drug from being available as a repeat prescription if a doctor or other prescriber stops or changes it.

Prescription and consumption of 'as required' drugs should be monitored with the same attention as regular medication. That is, a drug in this category should be revised in terms of the appropriateness of the drug, dosage/frequency and validity of the request.

There should be a secondary backup system to audit medication reviews. It should identify any patient who has not had a medication review within a reasonable period such as 12 months so that they can be recalled.

Patients should be encouraged to tell their GPs if they stop taking any regular medication, so that the practice repeat prescribing record can be amended accordingly.

No repeats should be given more than a few days in advance of the due date, unless there are exceptional circumstances. Practices should not supply further repeat prescriptions at shorter time intervals than have been authorised, without agreeing with the reason for an early request, e.g. the patient is going away on holiday and will not return before the next prescription is due. Reasons that might not be agreed include patients overusing their medication, patient convenience or the pharmacist 'owing' a patient an under-supply of medication. In the last case, the patient should return to collect the additional drug(s) rather than initiate an earlier request for the next repeat.

Practices should have a standard time limit for the collection of repeat prescriptions (for example seven working days), after which those not collected are destroyed. Practices should store repeat prescriptions awaiting collection in a secure way and determine that the person calling to collect the prescription is either the patient or a trusted representative of the patient.

A reliable staff member should transport repeat prescriptions to pharmacists nominated by the patient.

Prescribing qualifications

Doctors are able to prescribe so long as they are fully registered with the GMC and they demonstrate their fitness to practise on a regular basis, so that their professional qualifications are revalidated by the GMC every five years. Those who are provisionally registered can prescribe so long as they are supervised in doing so in a primary care setting.

District nurses and health visitors are qualified as part of their specialist practice training to prescribe from a limited nurse prescribing formulary. All nurses can now train to become extended formulary and supplementary prescribers through degree-level programmes, offered by many universities and colleges. Courses are commissioned and funded by Strategic Health Authority Workforce Development Directorates.[7] Supplementary prescribing is a new legal category of prescribing. An independent prescriber (e.g. a doctor) draws up a clinical management plan together with the supplementary prescriber. The clinical management plan can include any medication in the *British National Formulary*, except controlled drugs, and can be used for up to 12 months. The plan should list all drugs that the supplementary prescriber is likely to prescribe for a specified patient with a pre-diagnosed chronic condition. This means that it can include drugs for exacerbations or likely complications of the condition. Some useful examples of clinical management plans can be found on the Nurse Prescriber website.[8]

Nurses can also supply and administer drugs through patient group directions and patient-specific directions – both forms of written instructions from a doctor or dentist authorising the supply and administration of specific medicines.

Systems for nurses' prescribing, supply and administration of medicines need to be developed within a strict clinical governance framework to improve patient care and minimise risk to patient safety.

Case study 11.1 continued

The nurse practitioner who works in Richard's practice is mid-way through her supplementary prescribing qualification. Richard acts as her mentor, which requires tutorials and supervision. The practice also has plans to help the community physiotherapist train to use patient group directions to supply or administer medication now the regulations to allow them to do so are in place.[9]

Patient group directions (PGD) should be drawn up according to the legal requirements.[10–12] They are for prescription-only medicines for groups of patients who may not be individually identifiable before they present for treatment. This arrangement enables nurses to administer medication such as vaccines, or emergency contraception, so long as there is an appropriate PGD in place. To work in accordance with a PGD, a nurse must be named within the document and both the doctor giving his/her authorisation and the named nurse must sign it. The authorising doctor must be satisfied that the nurse is competent to administer the drug as described in the PGD. The information included in a PGD in a GP practice includes:

- the name of the GP practice
- the dates on which the PGD starts and expires
- a description of the medicine(s)
- the class of health professional who may supply or administer the medicine
- the signatures of the authorising doctor/nurse(s) to whom the PGD applies
- the clinical condition or situation
- a description of those patients excluded from treatment under the direction
- a description of circumstances necessitating further advice from the GP
- the arrangements for referral
- the details of dosage (including frequency, strength, quantity etc), and limits of the period over which the medicine should be administered
- relevant warnings including potential side-effects
- the follow-up arrangements.

Reaching a rationale about repeat prescriptions[3-5]

Prescribing should be rational and consistent. Practice prescribing formularies may help to establish such a culture, by creating opportunities for discussion between GP colleagues and local pharmacists. They should be able to reach consensus on systems for rational prescribing without limiting their clinical freedom unduly.[13] Rational prescribing focuses on efficacy and safety leading to successful clinical outcomes at reasonable cost.[14] There may be negative pressures on agreeing the rationale for a particular approach to prescribing, such as inappropriate pharmaceutical company marketing, patient expectations, poor GP organisation and fears of litigation.[14] On the other hand, training, peer support, local ownership of prescribing policy frameworks or guides and individual practitioners' willingness to change prescribing habits and receive feedback on their prescribing performance from the local prescribing advisor are all forces for good prescribing practice.[14]

Case study 11.1 continued

Richard and his GP partners decide to take benzodiazepines as an example drug to test out their repeat prescribing systems. They are already aware of the guidance by the Committee on Safety of Medicines (CSM) for the appropriate prescribing of benzodiazepines:

- two to four weeks for relief of severe or disabling anxiety that is subjecting the patient to unacceptable distress, or for severe or disabling insomnia in patients who are extremely distressed.
- *not* for the treatment of mild anxiety as long-term use exposes patients to risks such as road traffic accidents, dependence and falls.[3]

The reason that they picked out benzodiazepines was that they were aware that one-third of prescriptions for benzodiazepines nationally appeared to be for patients receiving long-term treatment.

  They audit the key procedures in their repeat prescribing of benzodiazepines. They find that only six patients are on long-term benzodiazepines and all have been reviewed in person within the previous nine months. All are long-established treatments and patients had not co-operated with reducing or replacing the drug. Their practice manager finds that it was possible for a member of the practice staff to illegally trigger a prescription for a patient and take it to a pharmacist, apparently on the patient's behalf while retaining it for personal use. The systems are re-organised to reduce the likelihood of such an event happening.

Monitoring repeat prescriptions[1,2]

There should be a practice monitoring system to check that defined review intervals are being followed and repeat prescribing systems are operating effectively. Pharmacists should have ready telephone access to GPs to discuss queries about patients' medication and particular prescriptions.

  It is good practice for GPs to take account of external feedback on their prescribing and systems. This may be by utilising feedback as Prescribing Analyses and Cost (PACT) or Scottish Prescribing Analysis (SPA) data,[3,14,15] by setting and comparing own practice with locally based criteria and standards,[16] welcoming the involvement of prescribing advisors or audit facilitators employed by PCOs. The PCO may have sophisticated electronic feedback of prescribing performance to compare with that of other local practices or national patterns. Community pharmacists will be increasingly involved in reviewing repeat prescribing as part of the enhanced services normally provided by accredited pharmacists in England.

GPs should be aware of the potential for fraud at every stage in the repeat prescribing process, and set up check systems to monitor that repeat prescriptions are being processed in a reliable way by ancillary staff and medical colleagues. This will be achieved by emphasising the need for continuous training/updating, and rotating staff members to ensure sharing of best practice and uniformity of standards of staff in the practice.[17]

Avoiding prescribing errors

About 660 million prescriptions are written each year in England by GPs. Around 1.8 million prescriptions are written by GPs and an estimated 0.5 million in hospitals in England everyday.[18] Defence societies report that there are about 200 claims involving medicines made against GPs each year.

Prescribing errors may occur at any stage in the decision-making process or in prescription writing. Reasons are:

- inadequate knowledge of the drug or the patient and their clinical condition
- illegible handwriting
- drug name confusion
- poor history taking
- calculation errors for size/age of patient
- the prescription is given to the wrong patient.

These type of errors can result in drugs being prescribed that are contra-indicated, or interact with others also being taken, or being prescribed at too high/low a dose for the patient's condition, or simply being wrong. One estimate of the frequency of preventable adverse drug events gave it as nearly 2% of all patients admitted to hospital, while another study of GP prescription errors averted by watchful pharmacists put the frequency of those errors as one in 10 000.

While adverse drug reactions should be reported to the Medicines and Healthcare products Regulator Agency (MHRA) of the Committee on Safety of Medicines on yellow cards (*see* the *British National Formulary*[3]), prescribing errors should be reported to the National Patient Safety Agency's (NPSA's) national reporting and learning scheme.[19] The remit of the NPSA is to collect, collate, review and analyse error reports. The NPSA produces and dissemi-nates solutions, so that those working in the NHS learn from errors, and so reduce risk.

Minimising opportunities for patients to abuse prescribed drugs

Patients may abuse prescribed drugs unintentionally. For example, taking caffeine- or codeine-containing analgesics for headache can trigger medication-overuse headaches. Taking some analgesics several times per week over a considerable time may cause, rather than relieve, headaches. Advise patients to restrict their use of this type of analgesic to no more than seven days per month.[20]

Some patients may intentionally request acute or repeat prescriptions of drugs that they want for a different reason from those for which they are prescribed. They may try it on, asking for replacement prescriptions explaining that they have lost the original prescription, accidentally spilled the contents of their bottle of tablets in a muddy puddle or that in a fit of pique or resolve they threw a whole bottle of tablets away in their refuse. If it has a street value, such as strong analgesics like diconal, hypnotics such as temazepam or other benzo-diazepines like diazepam, amphetamines such as dexamfetamine, or related drugs such as methylphenidate, they may be taking some of the medication themselves and selling part on.

Minimising opportunities for patients to abuse prescribed drugs, intention-ally or unintentionally, will depend on good organisation of regular reviews of medication, staying alert to which drugs might have a potential for abuse and only prescribing drugs that are justified by a patient's condition rather than triggered by a patient's request. When prescribing for patients who are being treated for drug misuse and dependence, guidelines on clinical management recommend that medical practitioners should not prescribe in isolation. They should liaise with others in a multidisciplinary team. Shared care with a local specialist is preferable, so that GPs have access to expert prescribing advice and guidance on medico-legal matters. No more than one week's drugs should be prescribed at a time, and particular care should be taken with induction on to any substitute medication, especially where self-reporting of the dosage is being relied upon.[21]

Good prescribing practice and the GMS contract[22]

You can achieve the 42 quality points on offer by establishing good prescribing protocols with systems to review medication. The points available are shown in Table 11.1.

Table 11.1:   Quality indicators for good prescribing practice

Indicator		Points
1	Details of prescribed medicines are available to the prescriber at each surgery consultation	2
2	The practice possesses the equipment and in-date emergency drugs to treat anaphylaxis	2
3	There is a system for checking the expiry dates of emergency drugs on at least an annual basis	2
4	The number of hours from requesting a prescription to availability for collection by the patient is 72 hours or less (excluding weekends and bank/local holidays)	3
5	A medication review is recorded in the notes in the preceding 15 months for all patients being prescribed four or more repeat medicines (standard: 80%)	7
6	The practice meets the PCO prescribing advisor at least annually and agrees up to three actions relating to prescribing	4
7	Where the practice has responsibility for administering regular injectable neuroleptic medication, there is a system to identify and follow up patients who do not attend	4
8	The number of hours from requesting a prescription to availability for collection by the patient is 48 hours or less (excluding weekends and bank/local holidays)	6
9	A medication review is recorded in the notes in the preceding 15 months for all patients being prescribed repeat medicines (standard 80%)	8
10	The practice meets the PCO prescribing advisor at least annually, has agreed up to three actions relating to prescribing and subsequently provided evidence of this	4
Total number of points for medicine management indicators		42

A list of sources of information in relation to appropriate prescribing is given at the end of the chapter.

Collecting data to demonstrate your learning, competence, performance and standards of service delivery

Example cycle of evidence 11.1

- Focus: prescribing practice (herbal medicines)
- Other relevant focus: communication

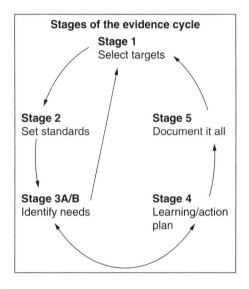

Stages of the evidence cycle

Stage 1
Select targets

Stage 2
Set standards

Stage 5
Document it all

Stage 3A/B
Identify needs

Stage 4
Learning/action plan

Case study 11.2

Mrs Down attends your surgery for review of her epilepsy with a smile on her face. She is obviously feeling much better than when she saw you last year when her depression was a problem. You check her drug records but she has only been on her regular carbamazepine. Her epileptic attacks seem well controlled and you quickly complete the stages in her epilepsy review according to the practice protocol. Just as she is leaving she mentions the benefits of the St John's Wort she has been taking for the last six months in helping her to feel so good. You ask her to sit down again and quiz her as to why she had not mentioned the drug before and checked it out with a doctor. Mrs Down is surprised you consider a herbal medicine like St John's Wort to be any of your business, so you explain about the interaction of St John's Wort with anti-epileptic drugs like carbamazepine.

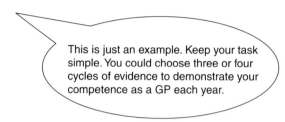

This is just an example. Keep your task simple. You could choose three or four cycles of evidence to demonstrate your competence as a GP each year.

Stage 1: Select your aspirations for good practice

The excellent GP:

- takes a full history about all drugs being taken by a patient whether prescribed or not prescribed
- knows what drugs commonly interact and where to access information about less common interactions.

Stage 2: Set the standards for your outcomes

Outcomes might include:

- the way learning is applied
- a learnt skill
- a protocol
- a strategy that is implemented
- meeting recommended standards.

- Be able to explain the risks and benefits of herbal medicines to patients.

Stage 3A: Identify your learning needs

- Ask the next 10 patients what they want to know about herbal medicines and reflect as to whether you can answer them knowledgeably.
- Visit the local health food shop and look at the array of herbal medicines for sale. Consider whether you are familiar with them and their properties or potential interactions.

Stage 3B: Identify your service needs

Any of the needs assessment exercises in 3A may also reveal service needs.

- Survey a number of patients attending your practice (e.g. 100) and ask them what herbal medicines they have taken in the previous year that they have bought from a shop or pharmacy. Provide prompts of names of commonly purchased herbal medicines (such as St John's Wort, glucosamine). Consider what you know about the effects of herbal medicines bought and taken by your patients.
- Ask the local pharmacist what herbal medicines your patients discuss with the pharmacist or counter staff. Find out if customers check the safety of the medications or enquire about purchase or interactions.
- Undertake a significant event audit where there is an interaction or potential interaction between a herbal medicine a patient is taking and a prescribed drug with adverse effects (e.g. the case study considered here). Consider in the analysis what factors might be preventable.

Stage 4: Make and carry out a learning and action plan

- Read up on the risks and benefits of herbal medicines and look at a website about herbal preparations.[23–25]
- Read up about the actions and benefits of St John's Wort.[3,26]
- Feed back to the practice team at an educational session what you have learnt about herbal medicines through work done in Stages 3 and 4. Invite the manager of a health food shop to join you to contribute his/her perspective. Decide on a rational consistent approach that the health professionals in the practice can adopt when advising patients about the risks and benefits of herbal medicines.

Stage 5: Document your learning, competence, performance and standards of service delivery

- Include your reflections on your reading about risks and benefits of herbal medicines.
- Keep notes of the significant event audit and any action plan for change.
- Include a memo from the in-house meeting about the practice approach when advising patients about risks and benefits of herbal medicines.

Case study 11.2 continued

Mrs Down was concerned that the St John's Wort she was taking might reduce blood levels of carbamazepine and so make a return of her epileptic fits more likely, especially as being a car driver is essential to her in her job as a courier. As her depression is better anyway, she agrees to stop the St John's Wort. If her depression returns in future, she will consult a GP if she decides she wants to try any other herbal medicine.

Example cycle of evidence 11.2

- Focus: generic prescribing
- Other relevant focus: relationships with patients

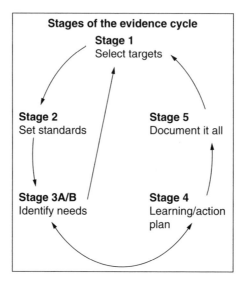

Stages of the evidence cycle

Stage 1
Select targets

Stage 2
Set standards

Stage 5
Document it all

Stage 3A/B
Identify needs

Stage 4
Learning/action plan

Case study 11.3

The pharmaceutical advisor urged Dr Count's practice to increase the proportion of drugs they prescribe generically yet again when he last visited the practice team. So this year, Dr Count is determined that they will do better as a partnership.

This is just an example. Keep your task simple. You could choose three or four cycles of evidence to demonstrate your competence as a GP each year.

Stage 1: Select your aspirations for good practice

The excellent GP:

- takes resources into account when choosing between treatments of similar effectiveness
- only prescribes treatments that make an effective contribution to the patient's overall management.

Stage 2: Set the standards for your outcomes

Outcomes might include:

- the way learning is applied
- a learnt skill
- a protocol
- a strategy that is implemented
- meeting recommended standards.

- Prescribe generically whenever there is a generic alternative drug except when bio-equivalence data prevents this.

Stage 3A: Identify your learning needs

- Review PACT (or SPA) data and compare your own prescribing perform- ance for generic prescribing with that of peers.
- Scrutinise a sheaf of prescriptions left out for signing, and check which of those with brand names have generic alternatives.
- Find out whether there is a reminder on the computer about drugs that, because there is difference in their bio-equivalence, must be prescribed by brand names.
- Ask the pharmacist to prompt you when you prescribe brand name drugs for which there is a generic alternative.

Stage 3B: Identify your service needs

Any of the needs assessment exercises in 3A may also reveal service needs.

- Ask for feedback by the prescribing advisor from your PCO about the best approach to generic prescribing.

- Undertake audits of generic prescribing, before and after the visit by the prescribing advisor from your PCO, to demonstrate progress. Action to increase generic prescribing will earn quality points (*see* page 194). Compare the proportions of generic prescribing per GP colleague for specific drugs.
- Collect feedback and comments from patients made to receptionists or local pharmacists, in relation to switching of their previously brand-named drugs to generic alternatives. Discuss whether the practice team needs to do more promotion to patients of why generic prescribing helps the health service.

Stage 4: Make and carry out a learning and action plan

- Arrange in-house discussions at least annually with the prescribing advisor from the PCO and other prescribing colleagues.
- Reflect on your PACT or SPA data and compare it with others.
- Read up about generic prescribing in a journal.

Stage 5: Document your learning, competence, performance and standards of service delivery

- Include successive quarterly printouts of your PACT or SPA data.
- Keep notes from the annual visits of the prescribing advisor, the action points and associated audits demonstrating the progress made on generic prescribing.
- Give examples of switches made from branded drugs to generic alternatives with anonymised patient records.

Case study 11.3 continued

The practice provides evidence that they have improved the proportion of drugs they prescribe generically by 10% over the course of six months, by an all out effort by each GP and with lots of prompting from the local pharmacist. This qualifies as one of the three actions taken relating to prescribing towards earning the eight possible quality points.

Example cycle of evidence 11.3

- Focus: relationships with patients
- Other relevant focus: clinical care

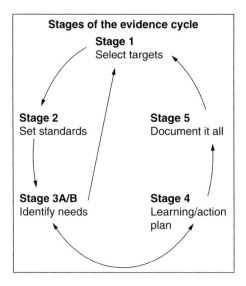

Stages of the evidence cycle

Stage 1
Select targets

Stage 2
Set standards

Stage 5
Document it all

Stage 3A/B
Identify needs

Stage 4
Learning/action plan

Case study 11.4

As Mr Blot leaves your consulting room, you realise that he is the third person that surgery who has neglected to take the tablets you have prescribed on a regular basis. Another patient's pregnancy was due to forgetting her contraception pill; Ms Garble's acne was not much better with the intermittent courses of antibiotics she takes and Mr Blot had just admitted that he only takes his low-dose aspirin 'when I remember it'.

This is just an example. Keep your task simple. You could choose three or four cycles of evidence to demonstrate your competence as a GP each year.

Stage 1: Select your aspirations for good practice

The excellent GP:

- involves patients in decisions about their care
- respects the rights of patients to refuse treatments
- gives patients the information they need about their problem, in a way they can understand.

Stage 2: Set the standards for your outcomes

Outcomes might include:

- the way learning is applied
- a learnt skill
- a protocol
- a strategy that is implemented
- meeting recommended standards.

- Be able to explain the options for drug therapy to patients so that they make informed decisions to take them.

Stage 3A: Identify your learning needs

- Write out a definition of concordance and check the description against a published view.[27]
- When you have given the patient a prescription, ask them a few more specific questions before they leave your consulting room. Ask if they would like any more information about side-effects, how to take the drug, what the drug does and what it's for, etc. Find out whether the patients still have information needs or are uncertain about proceeding to take the drug, even after you thought the decision to take a prescribed drug had been made.

Stage 3B: Identify your service needs

Any of the needs assessment exercises in 3A may also reveal service needs.

- Arrange for a survey of patients whereby someone relatively independent, such as a GP registrar, interviews patients and finds out in a non-threatening way whether they have adhered to the treatment regime prescribed by you and others in the practice. The interviewer should ask about reasons

for any non-compliance, and the extent to which the patients feel they were involved in the decision to prescribe the particular drugs.
- Advertise a 'drug amnesty' in your waiting room and at the local pharmacists. Advise patients that they can return any medicines that have not been taken. Look at what is returned and consider why patients have obtained drugs but not ingested them, before arranging for their destruction.

Stage 4: Make and carry out a learning and action plan

- Read up about concordance. Find out what information patients want and need about medicines, in publications like *Which* and other journals.[27,28]
- Visit your patient participation group or other patient-led group associated with the practice or PCO. Talk to the patient representatives about what else you can do to ensure concordance with patients.
- Stock up on literature for patients explaining about taking different types of medication. Download information from relevant websites.
- Try role-play with other colleagues interested in improving their skills in involving patients in decision making e.g. at a trainer's workshop. Play the doctor, the patient and observer roles. Critique each other and see how it feels to be the patient talking to a doctor who appears to 'know best'.
- Complete a rating scale for each of 10 consecutive consultations to determine the extent to which you are 'patient centred' or 'doctor centred'.[29] You might ask patients to complete the scale too and compare your perspectives and theirs.

Stage 5: Document your learning, competence, performance and standards of service delivery

- Include the completed rating scales of your patient centredness, with or without comparative views from patients.
- Keep notes of the role-play and how well you appeared to involve patients in decisions about their care (including prescribing decisions).
- Include examples of patient literature you have found to be helpful in informing patients.
- Include the survey and feedback results from patients, and your conclusions about what needs to be done.
- Keep copies of publications relating to concordance, and your reflections on how these apply to your own clinical practice.

> **Case study 11.4 continued**
>
> Your learning and service needs assessment exercises (*see* Stage 3 above) show that you do usually involve patients in decisions about prescribing. This is reinforced by the role-play and the rating scales. So, you keep on consulting in a patient-centred way, self-checking the way you practise so that you consistently involve patients in decisions about the options for their treatment.

References

1 Harris C and Dajda R (1996) The scale of repeat prescribing. *British Journal of General Practice*. **46:** 649–53.

2 Zermansky AG (1996) Who controls repeats? *British Journal of General Practice*. **46:** 643–7.

3 Joint Formulary Committee (2003) *British National Formulary*. British Medical Association/Royal Pharmaceutical Society, London.

4 Purves I and Kennedy J (1994) *The Quality of General Practice Repeat Prescribing*. Unpublished report to the Department of Health with supplementary report. Sowerby Foundation for Primary Care Information Research, Liverpool.

5 National Audit Office (1993) *Repeat Prescribing by General Medical Practitioners in England*. HMSO, London.

6 Audit Commission (1994) *A Prescription for Improvement*. HMSO, London.

7 Weedy S (2004) Right to prescribe. *NHS Magazine*. **February:** 10–11. www.nhs.uk/nhsmagazine/primarycare/archives/feb2004/newsfocus.asp

8 www.nurse-prescriber.co.uk

9 www.mhra.gov.uk

10 NHS Executive (2000) *Patient Group Directions (England)* HSC 200/026. NHSE, Leeds.

11 National Welsh Assembly (2000) *Review of Prescribing, Supply and Administration of Medicines by Health Professionals Under Patient Group Directions (PGD)*. National Welsh Assembly, Cardiff.

12 Scottish Executive Health Department NHS (2001) *Patient Group Directions*. www.show.scot.nhs.uk/sehd/mels/hdl2001_07.htm

13 Hastings A and McKinley R (1996) The development of a general practice formulary of drugs for out-of-hours care. *Pharmaceutical Journal*. **256:** 900–2.

14 Harrison I (1996) Prescribing facilitators can help. *Medical Interface*. **August:** 41–4.

15 Turner K (1997) Success for the quality in prescribing scheme. *Prescriber*. **January:** 65–6.

16 Bateman D, Eccles M, Campbell M *et al.* (1996) Setting standards of prescribing performance in primary care: use of a consensus group of general practitioners and application of standards to practices in the north of England. *British Journal of General Practice.* **46:** 20–5.

17 Department of Health (1997) *Prescription Fraud. An efficiency scrutiny.* Department of Health, London.

18 Department of Health (2004) Building a safer NHS for patients. Improving medication safety. Department of Health, London. www.dh.gov.uk/assetRoot/04/07/15/07/04071507.pdf

19 www.npsa.nhs.uk

20 Wakley G, Chambers R and Ellis S (2004) *Demonstrating Your Competence 3: cardiovascular and neurological conditions.* Radcliffe Publishing, Oxford.

21 Foord-Kelcey G (ed.) (2004) *Guidelines* vol 22. Medendium Group Publishing Ltd, Berkhamsted. www.eguidelines.co.uk

22 www.nhsconfed.org/gms

23 Ernst E (2001) Herbal medicinal products: an overview of systematic reviews and meta-analyses. *Perfusion.* **14:** 398–404.

24 Ernst E, Pittler MH, Stevenson C *et al.* (2001) *The Desktop Guide to Complementary and Alternative Medicine.* Mosby, Edinburgh.

25 http://medicines.mhra.gov.uk/ourwork/licensingmeds/herbalmeds/herbalsafety.htm

26 Linde K, Ramirez G, Mulrow CD *et al.* (1996) St John's Wort for depression: an overview and meta-analysis of randomised clinical trials. *British Medical Journal.* **313:** 253–8.

27 Elwyn G, Edwards A and Britten N (2003) 'Doing prescribing': how doctors can be more effective. *British Medical Journal.* **327:** 864–7.

28 Dickinson D and Raynor DKT (2003) What information do patients need about medicines? *British Medical Journal.* **327:** 861.

29 Tate P (2001) *The Doctor's Communication Handbook.* Radcliffe Medical Press, Oxford.

Sources of information in relation to appropriate prescribing

- *British National Formulary* www.bnf.org
- Department of Health, Drug Misuse and Dependence, Guidelines on Clinical Management 1999 www.dh.gov.uk/assetRoot/04/07/81/98/04078198. pdf
- Prodigy www.prodigy.nhs.uk

- Clinical Governance Research and Development Unit at the University of Leicester, audit protocol and data collection forms for prescribing in primary care www.le.ac.uk/cgrdu
- Medicines and Healthcare products Regulator Agency (MHRA), CSM, Freepost, London SW8 5BR. Tel: +44 (0)800 731 6789; http://medicines.mhra. gov.uk
- United Kingdom Medicines Information www.ukmi.nhs.uk

And finally

We hope that you have found that the stages in our 'cycle of evidence' are a useful approach to gathering information about what you need to learn. You can also use it to identify improvements you or others need to make to the way you deliver services.

It is easy to feel overwhelmed by the magnitude of the task to demonstrate that you are competent and perform consistently well as a doctor, in order to retain your licence to practise. Remember that you should be producing evidence about the breadth of your practice, every five years. Take your time and select three or four cycles of evidence each year, that span several headings of *Good Medical Practice* at one time.[1]

Ask others for help. Your practice manager or the receptionists should be able to help you to collect information about what you need to learn, or about gaps in services. You can delegate much of the administrative side. Your colleagues or your patients will be well placed to help you to set your aspirations for good practice and set achievable standards for your outcomes – of learning and improvements in service delivery. Perhaps your CPD tutor can help you to develop learning and action in your PDP. These cycles of evidence will be the nucleus of your PDP. Colleagues in the team can support you in documenting the evidence of your competence, performance and subsequent standards of service delivery. Other books in this series might help you to look at specific clinical areas, especially those where quality frameworks or special interests require your attention. Remember to visit this book's supporting website, which includes useful website links.[2]

So the evidence will be there ready to submit for appraisal interviews or revalidation, but the results will show what a good doctor you really are. This should give you increasing confidence and self-respect. Enjoy your professional glow.

References

1 General Medical Council (2001) *Good Medical Practice*. General Medical Council, London.

2 http://health.mattersonline.net

Index

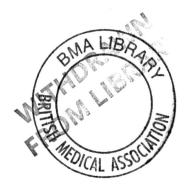